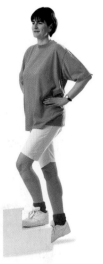

HEALTH AND HEALING
THE NATURAL WAY

DIET AND
WEIGHT CONTROL

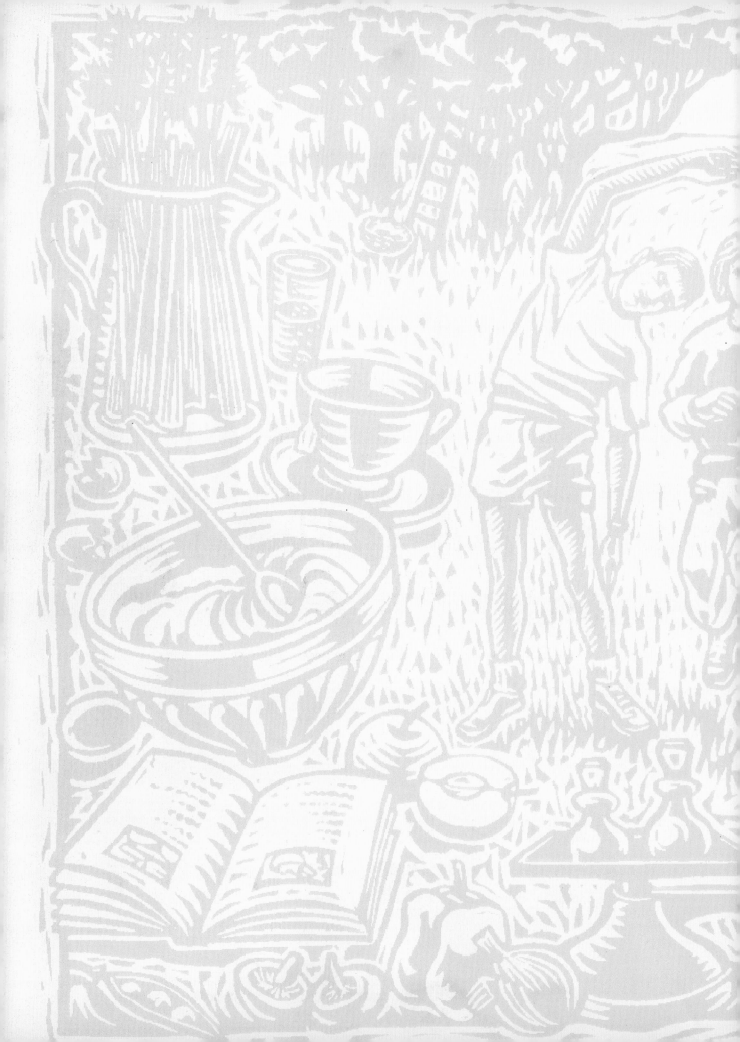

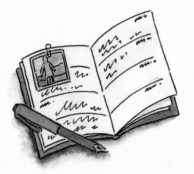

HEALTH AND HEALING
THE NATURAL WAY

DIET AND WEIGHT CONTROL

PUBLISHED BY

THE READER'S DIGEST ASSOCIATION LIMITED

LONDON NEW YORK SYDNEY MONTREAL CAPE TOWN

DIET AND WEIGHT CONTROL
was created and produced by
Carroll & Brown Limited
5 Lonsdale Road, London NW6 6RA
for The Reader's Digest Association Limited, London

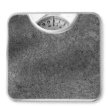

CARROLL & BROWN

Publishing Director Denis Kennedy
Art Director Chrissie Lloyd

Managing Editor Sandra Rigby

Editor Joanne Stanford
Assistant Editor Joel Levy

Art Editor Gilda Pacitti
Designer Jonathan Wainwright

Photographers Jules Selmes, David Murray

Production Christine Corton, Wendy Rogers

Computer Management John Clifford

First English Edition Copyright © 1997
The Reader's Digest Association Limited,
11 Westferry Circus, Canary Wharf,
London E14 4HE

Copyright © 1997
The Reader's Digest Association Far East Limited
Philippines Copyright © 1997
The Reader's Digest Association Far East Limited

ISBN 0 276 42264 3

Reproduced by Colourscan, Singapore
Printing and binding: Printer Industria Gráfica S.A., Barcelona

CONSULTANT

Dr Susan Jebb BSc, SRD, PhD
Head of Obesity Research, MRC Dunn Nutrition Centre

CONTRIBUTORS

Shirley Bond SRD
State registered dietitian and home economist

Tamsin Burnett-Hall
Home economist

Gary Frost BSc, SRD
State registered dietitian

Roger Newman-Turner BAc, ND, DO, MRO, MRN
Registered naturopath, osteopath and acupuncturist

Maria Pufulete
BSc Food Science

Claire Potter AFAA
Lifestyle planning and health and fitness consultant

Nicola Seabrook BSc, SRD
State registered dietitian

Carolyn Summerbell BSc, SRD
State registered dietitian

Nick Troop BSc, DHP
Psychologist in eating disorders

FOR THE READER'S DIGEST

Series Editor Christine Noble
Editorial Assistant Alison Candlin

READER'S DIGEST GENERAL BOOKS

Editorial Director Cortina Butler
Art Director Nick Clark

The information in this book is for reference only;
it is not intended as a substitute for a doctor's diagnosis and care.
The editors urge anyone with continuing medical problems
or symptoms to consult a doctor.

DIET AND WEIGHT CONTROL

More and more people today are choosing to take greater responsibility for their own health rather than relying on the doctor to step in with a cure when something goes wrong. We now recognise that we can influence our health by making an improvement in lifestyle – a better diet, more exercise and reduced stress. People are also becoming increasingly aware that there are other healing methods – some new, others very ancient – that can help to prevent illness or be used as a complement to orthodox medicine.

The series *Health and Healing the Natural Way* will help you to make your own health choices by giving you clear, comprehensive, straightforward and encouraging information and advice about methods of improving your health. The series explains the many different natural therapies now available – aromatherapy, herbalism, acupressure and many others – and the circumstances in which they may be of benefit when used in conjunction with conventional medicine.

The approach of DIET AND WEIGHT CONTROL is to emphasise that, despite the ever-growing slimming industry with its gimmicks, aids and miracle diets, there is really no replacement for eating the correct balance of the right foods and living an active life. The book sets out to dispel dieting myths and misleading messages about ideal body shape given out through the media. It discusses the true meaning of healthy body weight and the factors, physical and psychological, that influence your weight. You will find all the information necessary for you to assess your current weight and there is practical advice on how to take charge of your eating habits. If you are overweight or underweight for your height, setting a sensible weight target, reaching it and staying there, will both lower your risk of diseases such as coronary heart disease and increase your general health and well-being.

CONTENTS

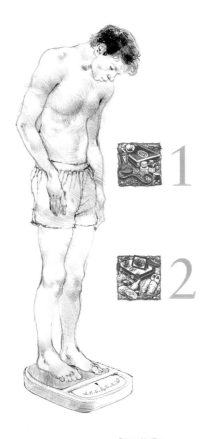

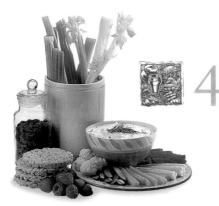
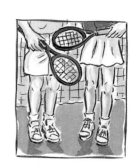

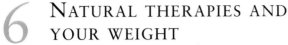
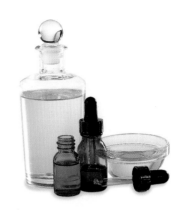

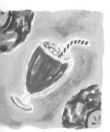

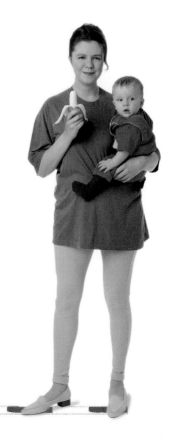

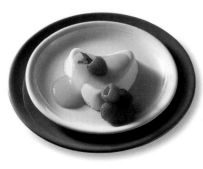
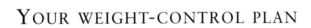

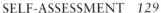

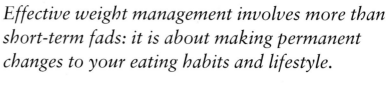

THE TRUTH ABOUT WEIGHT CONTROL

Effective weight management involves more than short-term fads: it is about making permanent changes to your eating habits and lifestyle.

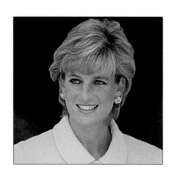

DIANA, PRINCESS OF WALES
Diana is well-known for having suffered from the chronic eating disorder, bulimia. She is now in good health, proving that the condition can be conquered.

BE REALISTIC!
Some people let the bathroom scales rule their life, looking almost daily for proof of weight reduction. Shedding pounds too quickly, however, is not healthy; a good weight-loss plan should advocate a weight loss of only about 0.5–1 kg (1-2 lb) a week.

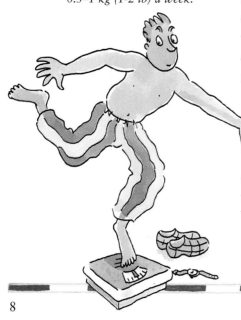

Even though Western society is becoming increasingly concerned about weight control, all the evidence points to the fact that we are far from successful at managing our weight. At one end of the spectrum eating disorders such as anorexia and bulimia are becoming more prevalent. At the other end people in Western societies are, on average, becoming increasingly overweight. The rate of obesity in the UK has more than doubled in the years between 1980 and 1994. Around 15 per cent of adults are obese and 50 per cent are overweight. Particularly worrying is the fact that obesity is increasing among children. Why is effective weight control such a problem today? And why do so many people find it so hard to achieve and maintain a healthy weight?

OUR MODERN LIFESTYLE

The answer lies in the changes in lifestyle and types of food available in Western countries over the past 60 years. Modern technology has reduced the amount of physical activity we perform in our daily lives at every level, from personal transport to labour-saving devices in the home and at work. The widespread availability of the car has had a dramatic effect on the average person's daily activity levels: even walking at a moderate pace burns 250 calories an hour, whereas driving only burns 100 calories an hour. At the same time, changes in social habits have meant that we're eating less structured meals, often bought ready-made from the supermarket or takeaways which are high in fat, supplemented with frequent high-calorie snacks. A recent study has revealed that up to 45 per cent of the average child's energy intake comes from snacks rather than from regular meals. This combination of high-fat foods with our increasingly sedentary lives is the principal reason for the steady weight gain recorded in countries such as Britain since the Second World War. The argument that lifestyle is primarily to blame is supported by the experience of immigrants from less wealthy countries coming to the affluent West. After a comparatively short time immigrant populations adopting the Western lifestyle show very similar patterns of diet-related problems, including obesity, to those found in the indigenous populations.

A more fundamental problem with weight control is inherent in basic human physiology. Our bodies are well designed to help us deal with starvation – in fact as we eat less our bodies become more and more efficient at functioning on less food. The metabolism slows down and we become more lethargic in order to conserve energy. This is why it is hard to continue losing weight by dieting alone: the body adapts to the change in energy intake and simply slows down all non-essential functions. The reason for this is that physiologically we are still hunter-gatherers, like our Stone Age ancestors. Our bodies are prepared for periods of semi-starvation, but when food is plentiful we are happy to continue to eat even if we are not actually physically in need of food. In the Stone Age, however, people led far more physical lives; constantly on the move and actively engaged in searching for food, they had energy needs far higher than that of the average desk worker today. In fact anthropologists draw direct correlations between the level of development of a society (with Stone Age societies at one end of the spectrum and industrialised ones like our own at the other) and the weight-related diseases and disorders from which it suffers. Diet and lifestyle are the factors that underlie this correlation.

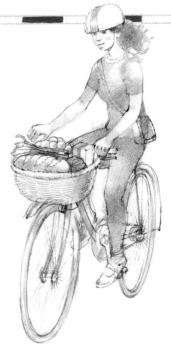

THE ROAD TO SUCCESS
Combining regular exercise and a healthy diet is the most successful way to lose weight. Exercise can be increased in simple ways such as walking or cycling when you would normally have used the car.

SO HOW DO YOU CONTROL WEIGHT?

Research has shown that in order to control weight properly we need to get the balance right in our daily lives between energy intake and energy expenditure. In other words, we need to make sure that we are eating the right amount of food for the amount of activity we perform daily. Our energy requirements are governed by a number of factors. To a large extent gender determines our fuel requirements: men tend to need to eat more than women because more of their body is muscle and muscle burns energy faster than fat. Energy requirements also change throughout our lives: children need more energy to support their growth, while adults need less as they get older and expend less energy. Then there are exceptional cases: athletes need to eat more food than the average person to sustain their high energy output. An athlete may burn in excess of

NATHAN PRITIKIN
The Pritikin diet, one of the most popular in recent years, was devised by Nathan Pritikin. Most nutritionists today, however, argue that the diet is too restrictive to be practical. Long-term weight control requires sustainable dietary changes.

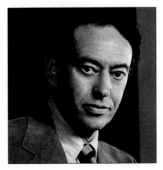

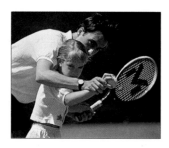

A HEALTHY START TO LIFE
It is important to encourage children to enjoy exercise by nurturing any interest they show in a particular sport.

4000 calories a day, whereas a sedentary man only needs around 2200 calories a day. Any increase in your level of activity will mean that your body burns more calories. Furthermore, regular sustained exercise can raise your metabolic rate, meaning that your body uses more energy in every activity you do from breathing to playing sport.

It is also important to look at the type of food you're eating. Weight control isn't simply about restricting food, it's about getting the right balance of food in your diet. The good news here is that eating healthily by reducing the amount of fat and eating more complex carbohydrates and fruit and vegetables is also a successful plan for weight control. Research has shown that complex carbohydrates – breads, pasta and grains – are the body's preferred source of energy. Dietary fat, on the other hand, tends to be simply stored by the body.

AREN'T THERE ANY SHORTCUTS?

Strict dieting can often produce rapid weight loss, and many people sign up for a variety of programmes and classes, often based around meal substitutes, to get results in just weeks. But the vast majority of people who lose weight in this way simply regain it over the following months. People who make a habit of this – whose weight is constantly 'yo-yoing' – may be doing themselves more harm than good, both physically and mentally. For example, slimmers who quickly regain all the weight they have lost often feel guilty and then depressed by their failure to keep to the diet.

Other people turn to clinics offering cosmetic surgery or drug treatment. A variety of cosmetic procedures are available, from liposuction to surgical intervention in the gut designed to prevent or reduce eating, or inhibit the digestion or absorption of food. The drugs used may have side effects and can currently only be prescribed for a limited period of time. Such treatments are extreme and recommended only for people whose health is in immediate danger because of a weight problem.

The potential market for a drug that would 'cure' obesity and reduce anyone's weight is huge, and pharmaceutical companies invest heavily in research into the biology of eating, appetite and weight control. But despite many exciting discoveries, from the role of hormones to the discovery of a gene that appears to control obesity in mice (the *ob* gene), the overwhelming message to emerge from research is that the causes of human weight problems are too

HOME-GROWN GOODNESS
Growing your own fruits and vegetables will ensure you always have something fresh and flavoursome for the table. It will save you money, give you great satisfaction and can also be good exercise.

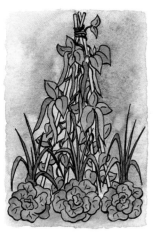

complex to be isolated to a single factor. This means that there is not, and is unlikely to be, a 'magic pill' that can be taken to help us banish fat and shed weight without any conscious effort.

Nutritionists agree that the only really successful way of losing weight is a general improvement in diet and activity, an approach taking into account your whole lifestyle. The benefits can include more energy, better sleep and a range of improvements to general health and well-being from lower blood pressure to enhanced self-confidence.

DO YOU NEED TO CHANGE YOUR WEIGHT?

Most people, particularly women, immediately answer yes to this question, but it is important to give your answer more careful thought. As a first step you need to accurately measure your weight in relation to your height and frame. The most respected method for doing this is the Body Mass Index (BMI) system (see page 25). Establishing your BMI will tell you whether you are underweight, of average weight, overweight or obese. You can then make a sensible decision about the degree to which you need to change your weight.

Knowing exactly why you want to diet is important if you are to set realistic goals for yourself. The best reason to lose weight is for your health. Being obese (having a BMI of over 30) is a major risk factor for a variety of disorders including heart disease, diabetes and some cancers. Obesity also has a detrimental effect on self-esteem and confidence and many obese people suffer from depression.

But some people who are overweight rather than obese, or who may even be of normal weight, see losing weight as a way to solve all the other things they are unhappy about in their lives. Problems at work, with partners or other family members can all be blamed on their excess weight. Weight loss cannot provide a magical solution to other problems in your life, and if this is an underlying cause of wanting to lose weight it is important to try to examine more closely the reasons behind why you're unhappy with your life. Trying to lose weight for reasons like these is a serious risk factor for some eating disorders. Studies show that the instance of bulimia, for example, trebled between 1988 and 1993. The psychological aspects of weight are discussed in Chapter 2. Finally, many people, especially young women, are strongly influenced by the media and its obsession with slim models. Fashions change, however, and women who in

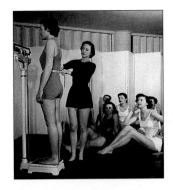

THE DIETING FASHION
Since the Second World War women have become increasingly obsessed about weight, often without cause. These women, all within healthy weight for their age and height, are being persuaded to lose extra pounds on a three-week health and beauty course.

HERE'S TO YOUR HEALTH
A diet should be undertaken with care. Some strict diets are lacking in the vitamins and minerals found in fresh fruits and vegetables which are essential for good health.

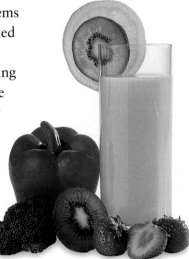

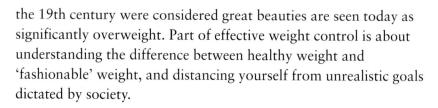

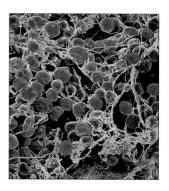

THE ROLE OF ADIPOSE
Fat cells (the brown and red rounded cells shown above) are held within adipose tissue in the body. Dietary fat which has not been burned off by the body is stored in these cells.

CUTTING BACK ON FAT
Trimming fat from chops and bacon before cooking can significantly reduce your fat intake. Before serving meat, blot off excess fat with kitchen paper.

the 19th century were considered great beauties are seen today as significantly overweight. Part of effective weight control is about understanding the difference between healthy weight and 'fashionable' weight, and distancing yourself from unrealistic goals dictated by society.

SUSTAINABLE WEIGHT CONTROL

Diet and Weight Control covers all these issues from first principles to practical tips. It discusses normal body shape and size, the factors that influence weight, and practices that can be adopted to manage and reduce weight.

Chapter 1 contrasts the pressures imposed by the media on people's self-image with the truth about what is a normal and healthy body shape. It explains how to tell if you are really overweight (or underweight) and if you need to take action. Chapter 2 discusses the physical and psychological factors that influence and determine your weight. Emerging discoveries in the fields of genetics, hormones and pharmaceutical research are covered, together with the basic anatomy, physiology and psychology of appetite and eating. Chapter 3 presents a general overview of how to manage your weight, looking at why we eat too much or too little, and what we should eat to stay healthy throughout our lives. Chapter 4 explains the details of how different types of food affect weight.

Chapters 5, 6 and 7 cover, respectively, the theories and practices of exercise, natural therapies, and diet with regard to weight control. Each chapter discusses the elements involved and the practical steps you can take for yourself, including advice on how to involve your whole family, old and young. Chapter 8 presents a fully integrated personal weight-control plan that you can adapt to your own needs and goals, with tips on how to fit a healthy diet which fulfills the needs of both you and your family into a busy schedule. Menus and recipes in Chapter 9 show you how to apply the principles of low-fat cooking to your own meal planning. Throughout the book special sections describe the role of different professionals in the field of diet and weight control, while selected case studies illustrate some common problems that can arise and how to deal with them. *Diet and Weight Control* offers no crash diets or miracle methods. Instead it clearly sets out the basic tenets of achievable, sustainable weight control for a healthier, happier life.

How much do you know about weight control?

There are many misconceptions in the field of weight control and dieting. Even the most simple task of estimating exactly how much you eat during the day is difficult to do accurately. You may be surprised about just how much fat and sugar you consume from processed foods. And many people are unaware of the health benefits that simple lifestyle changes, such as walking up the stairs instead of taking the lift, can bring in the long term.

Q WOULD YOU LIKE TO LOSE 5 kg (11 lb) IN TWO WEEKS?
If you answered 'yes', then you're probably making a serious mistake. Diet regimes that produce such dramatic effects usually make you eat a severely unbalanced diet, and the weight reduction you achieve is more from fluid and protein loss than from shedding fat. This is not a healthy approach, and the weight is likely to be quickly regained when you stop the diet and resume normal eating patterns. See Chapter 7.

Q DO YOU FIND IT IMPOSSIBLE TO RESIST FATTY FOODS?
Research shows that most people find fatty foods more tasty and filling than other types of foods. Some theorists argue that this reflects our Stone Age past: for our Neolithic ancestors fat was a rare and potentially life-saving treat. Today we have to work hard to overcome our evolutionary predisposition for fatty foods, and *Diet and Weight Control* provides a wealth of tips and food ideas, from snacks to full menus, to help you do just that. See Chapters 4 and 9.

Q DO YOU LOOK AT FOOD LABELS?
Many people don't check the calorie and fat content of the foods they buy and yet surprising discoveries can be made by doing this. Learning which foods are a healthy buy is an important part of a weight-control plan. Chapter 4 looks into the value of 'health foods', shows you how to calculate the fat content of foods, and includes a calorie and fat content chart of popular foods. The 'cutting calories' boxes in every chapter will also help you to make healthy food choices.

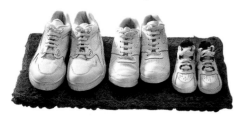

A FAMILY COMMITMENT
Every member of the family will benefit from increasing their level of exercise and it is especially important for children in today's computer-game age. Make the outdoors fun for children by exercising as a family; playing football in the park and going on walks or cycle rides will all provide good aerobic activity.

SCHOOL LUNCHES
Encourage children to adopt healthy eating habits from an early age. Try to include fresh fruit in their daily packed lunch rather than a snack like chocolate or cake. Include a treat once in a while, but remember that a sweet tooth gained at this age is likely to stay with them to adulthood.

Q DO YOU HAVE A SEDENTARY JOB?

Scientists link rising rates of obesity to two factors. One is the changing diet of modern society. The other is the steady decline in levels of physical activity. Automation and labour-saving devices mean many people now lead a more sedentary life, especially if they work in jobs where they sit all day. Even modest changes to your routine, like getting off the bus two stops from home and walking the rest of the way, can radically improve your activity levels. Every small change you make will help with losing weight and sustaining that reduction, while at the same time improving your health and well-being. Chapter 5 describes the ways in which you can bring exercise into your life. 'Quick fitness tips' in every chapter offer easy-to-implement advice on increasing your day-to-day activity levels, while 'burning off calories' boxes explain various forms of exercise and the muscle groups targeted by each one.

Q DO YOU FIND MOST LIFESTYLE ADVICE TOO UNREALISTIC TO ASPIRE TO?

Sweeping statements about the need to change your lifestyle and to replace your normal diet with one of bran and pulses are not very helpful. Most people do not want to become wholefood vegetarians or fitness fanatics, while others may be concerned about the expense of organic foods and supervised exercise classes. The personal weight-control plans in Chapter 8 will help you to set realistic goals, and offer advice on how to solve common lifestyle problems.

Q DOES YOUR FAMILY SABOTAGE YOUR HEALTHY EATING INTENTIONS?

Many people find that their family can make weight-control plans difficult to implement. Children especially can be fussy eaters and reject the change to healthy, low-fat foods. Chapter 3 looks at the different food needs of children and adults, and shows you how to ensure that children receive the right level of nutrition without compromising your own low-fat approach. The recipes in Chapter 9 will give you ideas on adapting family meals, making them low in fat but high in flavour and nutrients. There are also more creative recipes that may help to persuade a reluctant partner that dietary change not only makes health sense but can also be delicious.

CHAPTER 1

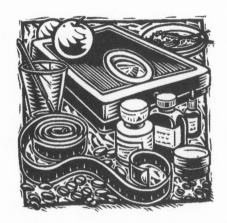

IS YOUR WEIGHT HEALTHY?

*The decision to begin a weight-loss programme
needs to be taken with care. Assessing the reasons
why you are unhappy with your weight, examining
your general health and well-being, and recognising
a distinction between your own body shape
and unrealistic images promoted by society,
are important first steps to take.*

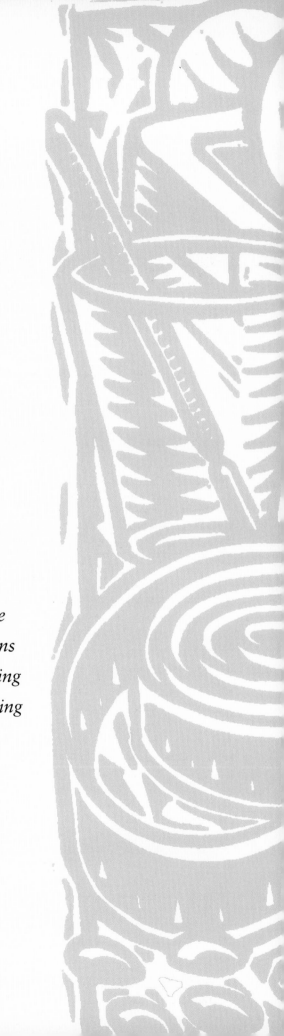

HEALTHY WEIGHT

Ideal weight can be defined in two ways. Firstly in terms of attractiveness, and secondly in terms of health. The two definitions do not necessarily mean the same thing.

It is important to recognise the extent to which our perception of ideal weight is influenced by fashion, advertising and the media. The images presented to society are not always representative of recognised healthy body weight statistics and can sometimes be startlingly different. Make sure that your weight goal is realistic, and not just an idea of how you would like to look – an attempt to attain an unrealistic body shape is bound to fail and may even be dangerous.

IMAGE AND WEIGHT

The ideal 'attractive' body image changes over time and varies between cultures. In the West at present the favoured shape is thin and there has been a great deal of speculation as to why this should be so.

Since the 1950s there has been a marked increase in leisure time, travel and outdoor pursuits. Many fashion commentators feel that activities such as swimming, tennis and travel, once restricted to the privileged classes, have been responsible for promoting the slim look as women strive to attain a figure suitable for public display at the beach, pool or gym. Others argue that society has come to associate desirability with youth. The slim, adolescent figure has become the ideal, and models as young as 15 set the standards for the ideal figure. The fashion industry has been blamed for preferring their clothes to be modelled on very thin models. Designers argue back that clothes simply look better on a thin, broad-shouldered body type and that they are committed to marketing their designs in the most effective way possible.

Whatever the reasons behind society's fixation with slimness, the idea is reinforced in almost every aspect of daily life through advertising and the media. Images of flat-stomached, adolescent girls seen on billboards and buses, and in magazines, television and film, sell everything from holidays to cheese. Subconsciously, we receive the message that being thin will make us more desirable, successful and happy.

But fashions can change. The history of Western art shows that up until very recently ideal female beauty was represented by significantly rounder women. Today the Venus de Milo would be considered to have large thighs and to be in need of some tummy firming exercises. Rubens' nudes are even more voluptuous, and Renoir's women are uniformly plump.

WHAT IS NORMAL?

What was considered ideal body weight used to be derived from charts published by the American Metropolitan Life Insurance Company. The company calculated the lowest mortality associated with a particular weight for a given height, based on the medical records of the company's clients. From this data they drew up optimum weights for people of all heights, but these charts have changed significantly since they first appeared in the 1920s. It was realised that the original samples were unrepresentative, and optimum weights have gradually been increasing over the past few decades.

Today the most respected method for assessing weight is the Body Mass Index (BMI), calculated by dividing your weight

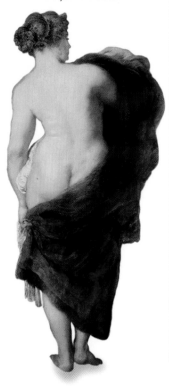

CHANGING TIMES
This detail taken from Rubens' Judgement of Paris *shows how much society's perception of human beauty has changed over the years. Today, this figure would be deemed too overweight to be fashionable.*

DID YOU KNOW?
In many countries plumpness is considered attractive. The Chinese associate a full figure with prosperity and longevity and in many Arab countries it is symbolic of fertility and womanhood. In these cultures being plump not only symbolises beauty but also conforms to the stereotype of the caring, reliable mother.

THE CHANGING IMAGE OF IDEAL BODY WEIGHT

The fashion industry's image of ideal body weight has changed dramatically through the years and is becoming increasingly unrealistic. For the majority of ordinary women, this perceived ideal shape is a physical impossibility.

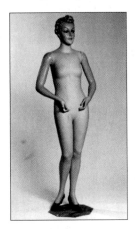

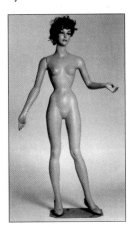

1930 VERSUS 1960
A study by the University Central Hospital in Helsinki, Finland, found that before the 1950s the calculated percentage of 'body fat' shown on mannequins was within a desirably healthy range. Since the 1950s, however, they have gradually become too thin to be representative of a healthy weight. By 1960 (right) impossibly narrow waists and hips and thin thighs had replaced the more realistic pear-shape of the 1930s (left). Unfortunately, the 1960 figure is still in vogue today.

in kilograms by your height in metres squared (see page 25). Optimum BMIs are arrived at by measuring mortality against weight for height. Even though mortality risks vary from country to country, it is possible to say that the optimum BMI for both men and women is between 20 and 25. Individuals with a BMI greater than 30 are classified as obese and should lose weight for the benefit of their health.

If your BMI is within the appropriate range for your weight and height but you still want to improve your shape, exercises targeted to tone the particular part of the body you are unhappy with may be more worthwhile than trying to lose weight.

WEIGHT AND THE INDIVIDUAL

Optimum weight for an individual may vary over time. There are many physiological changes that affect weight during a lifetime (see Chapter 2), and for women there are the added effects of the menstrual cycle, pregnancy and the menopause.

From birth to childhood

As there is little data on how weight gain during the early years of life relates to long-term health, it is difficult to give precise healthy weight figures for children. But it is important to monitor your child's growth and health so that you can identify when weight problems are sufficiently severe to warrant seeking medical advice. The chart overleaf shows average growth rates from birth to adolescence. However, since children differ in their genetic potential for growth, a group of normal children of the same age will vary in weight and height. But a normal child should not be greatly dissimilar to other children of the same age – if you feel any cause for concern discuss it with your doctor.

With obese children, it is important to ensure that they have a healthy balanced diet which maintains a constant weight. This will allow normal growth to continue whereas more severe measures to produce weight loss can interfere with this process. As the child gains height, they should effectively 'grow into their weight'.

From adolescence to adulthood

Weight and height increases at a steady rate throughout childhood until the onset of puberty, when there is a sudden growth spurt. Extra food is required at this time to fuel the development of muscle, bone and other tissues. This growth spurt continues until the late teens when bone growth tails off and little extra muscle is put on, unless muscle building exercise is carried out.

Girls lay down extra fat in adolescence which is distributed to help develop female characteristics like fuller breasts and rounded hips. Some adolescents put on extra weight due to a sedentary lifestyle; this may lead to a weight problem that lasts into adulthood unless steps are taken to exercise regularly while following a healthy, balanced diet.

SOCIAL RULES
The fashion world's obsession with the 'super-waif' figure, and the subsequent media saturation, has been directly linked to the increase in eating disorders seen in much of the developed world.

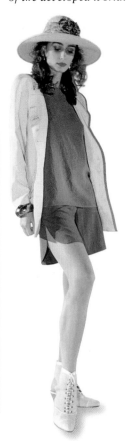

HEALTHY WEIGHT GAIN DURING PREGNANCY

During pregnancy you should put on some weight for the benefit of both yourself and the baby. The following figures are a guide to how much additional weight you should be aiming for dependent upon your BMI (see page 25) at conception:

▶ *Underweight with a BMI below 19.8: 12.5–18 kg (2 st–2 st 12 lb)*

▶ *Normal weight with a BMI of 19.8–26: 11.5–16 kg (1 st 11 lb–2 st 7 lb)*

▶ *Overweight with a BMI of 26–29: 7–11.5 kg (1 st 1 lb–1 st 11 lb)*

▶ *Obese with a BMI over 30: at least 6 kg (13¼ lb)*

AVERAGE WEIGHTS FOR CHILDREN (kg)

This growth table helps you monitor and record the development of your child from baby to teenager. It shows the expected weight for healthy, average children and will alert you to possible irregularities at an early stage in their development.

AGE	Birth	6–12 m	1–2 y	3–4 y	5–6 y	7–8 y	9–10 y	11–12 y	13–14 y	15–16 y	17–18 y
BOYS	3–4	6	12	16	20	24	29	35	45	58	64
GIRLS	3–4	6	12	16	20	24	29	37	50	56	58

Pregnancy and breastfeeding

Pregnancy is a period of considerable metabolic and nutritional change. Many people naturally assume that a mother needs a lot of additional energy to support her new lifestyle, and to meet the demands placed on her body by the rapid growth of her baby, the placenta and other new tissues of pregnancy. But whether or not a pregnant women actually needs this extra energy intake is a matter for debate.

Recent studies have revealed that there is an extraordinary range in the way women's bodies respond to pregnancy. Some women lay down huge amounts of body fat while others gain very little. Some experience a significant increase in their metabolic rate (see page 29), therefore using more energy than before they became pregnant, while others have a lower rate. These changes only last while the woman is pregnant and seem to be part of the body's way of sensing how well-nourished a woman is and then responding by providing the best conditions for the growing baby.

During pregnancy, you should eat as much or as little as your appetite tells you but you should consult your doctor if you put on excessive weight or very little weight in relation to your body mass index figure (see left). Women who gain a lot of weight are at higher risk of having complications during pregnancy, and are more likely to retain the extra weight afterwards. In contrast, women who gain very little weight have a higher risk of having low birth weight or premature babies. Women should not diet during pregnancy as it can be dangerous. There is evidence that severe dieting may limit the growth of the baby and ultimately be responsible for a low birth weight baby. Severe dieting during breastfeeding will also take a toll on the mother's health and may cause a decrease in milk production.

EXERCISING SAFELY DURING PREGNANCY

Regular exercise during pregnancy will help you to retain muscle tone, prevent build up of fat and can also help to ensure a smooth, less painful birth. Devise an exercise programme after consultation with your doctor and then put aside a set time, at least three times a week, to exercise. Always warm up thoroughly before exercising by stretching all your muscles and ensure you take time to cool down and relax afterwards.

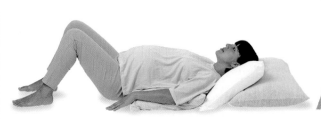

EXERCISING THE PELVIC FLOOR MUSCLES
These muscles cradle and protect the womb. Lie flat on your back with knees bent. Squeeze your pelvic muscles, as if to stop a flow of urine, hold for 10 seconds and repeat 10 times.

RELAXATION
Thoroughly relaxing after exercise is vital. Lying flat on your back with your legs raised on a bed or chair is especially relaxing and is particularly good for swollen ankles and feet.

THE MENOPAUSE AND WEIGHT GAIN

Women may experience slight weight gain after menopause. This is due in part to the slowing of the metabolism, but mostly it is just a by-product of the ageing process and a decrease in physical activity. More pronounced, however, is the change in fat distribution: after menopause, fat is deposited around the stomach. This occurs as a result of reduced levels of oestrogen in the body.

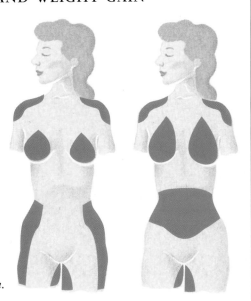

FAT REDISTRIBUTION
Before the menopause (left) fat is distributed around the buttocks and thighs, as well as the shoulders and breasts. After menopause (right), fat tends to collect around the front of the stomach, on the breasts and about the abdomen.

Middle age

People tend to get fatter as they get older and many people complain of 'middle-age spread'. There is a small decline in the body's metabolic rate from about the age of 30 (approximately 2 per cent for each subsequent decade), but more significant is the marked decrease in physical activity that commonly occurs in this age group. Active participation in sport steadily declines with age, and more time is spent watching television – if energy intake is not reduced in proportion weight will be gained.

At the same time muscle cells become weaker (atrophy) and there is a shift in the body's overall ratio of muscle to fat; there tends to be more fatty tissue and less lean. Exercising regularly will help to slow down muscle atrophy and prevent the build up of fat, so you need to maintain or even increase your level of physical activity as you get older. This may mean that you need to find new activities that are easily fitted into daily routines. Walking 30 minutes each day, for example, could improve your health and help to control your weight.

Menopause

The question whether the menopause alters women's body weight or not remains a controversial one. While many women would claim that they put on weight during the menopause, most studies demonstrate that this can be accounted for by the simple fact that people tend to gain weight as they get older anyway, suggesting that age and not the menopause is responsible for the increase. However, the menopause is associated with changes in fat distribution (see above). Some women who have been prescribed hormone replacement therapy (HRT) to help relieve the symptoms of the menopause believe that the treatment is the cause of their weight gain, but there is no conclusive evidence to support this claim.

Old age

By the age of 70, many people's bodies will have about twice as much fat as in their 30s and only half as much muscle tissue. Keeping active will help to preserve muscle tissue and help maintain a desirable weight, but being slightly overweight in old age is associated with only modest health risks. This is

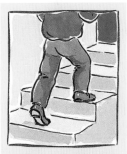

QUICK FITNESS TIP
Taking the stairs instead of the lift will burn a few calories and help to tone your leg muscles.

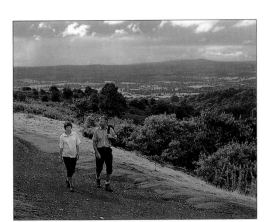

MAINTAINING FLEXIBILITY
Many older people suffer from joint problems such as arthritis as they age and become less active. Light aerobic exercise such as walking, swimming, or ballroom dancing will help to prevent the joints from becoming too stiff and will boost the body's energy expenditure.

a time to avoid extremes. Thinness is a major risk factor for hip fractures associated with osteoporosis, while obesity will increase the risk of, or even exacerbate, diseases such as diabetes, heart disease and hypertension.

CAN YOU BE TOO THIN?

Many people aspire to be thin but it is vital to realise that, contrary to the image increasingly portrayed in fashion and the media, thinness does not always mean you are fit and healthy. Being underweight can place as many physical and psychological strains on the body as being overweight.

Health risks of being underweight

As someone loses weight, typical symptoms such as fatigue and lethargy appear. These are part of the body's natural response to starvation; the body conserves energy by decreasing the energy output involved in all voluntary physical activity.

In children, being underweight can stunt growth and delay puberty – problems that can be irreversible. It is therefore vital that children are given a healthy, balanced diet and discouraged from any form of dieting. If you notice that your child is losing weight you should consult your doctor.

In women, being underweight can cause menstrual and fertility problems; below a certain weight women do not menstruate at all and are infertile. Older women who are too thin tend to suffer more from osteoporosis, and there may be some justification for doctors recommending postmenopausal women to be slightly plump rather than too thin. The risk of ill-health increases below a BMI of 19 (see page 25). A BMI of less than 12 is generally fatal. If you are seriously underweight, for example your BMI is less than 16, or if you are losing weight without trying and the reason is hard to pinpoint, consult your doctor, as it may be a sign of an underlying problem.

Causes of being underweight

There are a number of reasons for being underweight; some are straightforward, others are more complex.

A disorder of the thyroid gland, which helps to regulate the body's energy levels, can lead to the overproduction of thyroid hormones. This condition is called hyperthyroidism (see page 34) and can produce a range of symptoms including weight loss.

Food allergies and intolerances can also cause weight loss. Many food intolerances produce symptoms such as indigestion and nausea which reduce appetite. An intolerance to gluten can lead to coeliac disease, characterised by diarrhoea and weight loss.

Any physical illness that includes trauma, inflammation, infection, or repair to tissues can cause weight loss mainly because of a decrease in appetite. With appropriate care, weight loss can be prevented or at least minimised. Sometimes it is possible to identify a specific cause, such as drugs causing nausea or vomiting, but often the cause is difficult to pinpoint. If you suffer from loss of appetite consult your GP or a dietitian.

Stress and depression can also lead to a loss of appetite and to digestive problems such as nausea and irritable bowel syndrome which can in turn reduce appetite. Stress and depression may, however, signal deeper emotional problems which in extreme cases may lead to the eating disorders anorexia nervosa and bulimia nervosa (see page 39). Anorexia nervosa is characterised by severe weight loss which can be fatal. Bulimia sufferers tend not to show such extreme weight loss as sufferers of anorexia, but they may still be underweight. Repeated vomiting can lead to other health problems too (see page 42).

Gaining weight

The best way to gain weight is to increase the size and number of meals you consume, and their nutrient density. If you have been underweight for a significant period, however, your body may find it difficult to cope with large amounts of food at any one time. It is usually advisable to start by gradually increasing the frequency of meals every day over a few weeks.

Your weight gain plan needs to be well thought out. It is important to keep the balance of food right and not be tempted by high-fat, calorie-laden foods in the hope of putting on weight quickly. You can eat healthily and still increase your calorie intake – make sure you eat a good mixture of starchy foods such as bread, pasta and potatoes, fruit and vegetables, and a moderate amount of protein and dairy foods to maintain the right balance of vitamins, minerals, protein and fibre necessary for good health. High-fat and sugary foods, as for any diet, should be eaten in moderation.

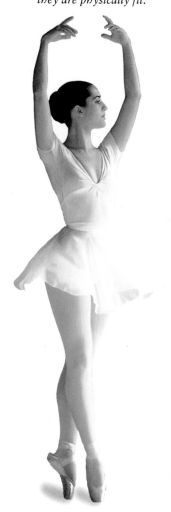

MUSCLE POWER
Ballet dancers are typically very thin so how do they stay healthy at such a low weight? The answer is that a disproportionate amount of their body weight is highly toned muscle, and they are physically fit.

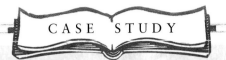

The Diabetes Sufferer

Diabetes that develops in adult life is known as non-insulin-dependent because it can usually be treated without requiring injections of insulin. Although insulin production is normal, the tissues of the body become unresponsive to it and typical diabetic symptoms ensue. Being overweight compounds the problem as high levels of fatty tissue further reduces the effect of insulin.

Mary is a 64-year-old retired factory worker with a fairly sedentary lifestyle and a weight problem. She skips breakfast but snacks all day, preferring fried foods and meat to salads and grills. Recently she has noticed that she has been tiring more easily, particularly in the morning, and has found herself going to the toilet more often while also feeling very thirsty all the time. She became really worried when she had a dizzy spell, followed by blurred vision and a feeling of numbness in her hands and legs. She went to see her doctor, who diagnosed her as having adult-onset, or non-insulin-dependent, diabetes. He not only prescribed her a course of drug treatment, but also referred her to a nutritionist.

WHAT SHOULD MARY DO?

Non-insulin-dependent diabetes can often be controlled through diet. To achieve this, Mary must first exclude sugar from her diet and replace it with a steady supply of complex carbohydrates which will balance the glucose levels in her blood. She also needs to consume more soluble fibre to regulate her body's absorption of carbohydrates. The nutritionist recommends that she should never skip a meal and to replace her sugary snacks with healthy options like vegetable crudités or fruit. For her main meals she should use beans and pulses – especially lentils – as a base for high fibre, low-fat meals. This healthier eating programme will also help her to lose weight.

Action Plan

DIET
Eat beans, pulses, fruit and vegetables for fibre and carbohydrates. Brewer's yeast is a good source of chromium and thiamine (to help prevent hand and foot numbness).

HEALTH
Seek medical advice. Treatment may be with drugs followed by a consultation with a nutritionist to introduce new eating habits.

EATING HABITS
Eat regular, evenly spaced meals, and completely exclude sugary snacks from the diet, replacing them with complex carbohydrates.

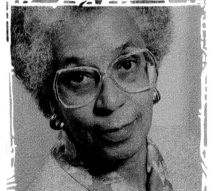

DIET
Missing out on complex carbohydrates, fibre and vital minerals like chromium and zinc worsens diabetic symptoms.

EATING HABITS
Skipping meals can lower blood sugar to dangerous levels.

HEALTH
Diabetes can be very dangerous if left untreated, leading to heart disease, kidney and eye problems and neurological disorders.

HOW THINGS TURNED OUT FOR MARY

Although she found it hard to give up her sweets, Mary did change her diet and by eating regular, healthy meals has weaned herself off drugs, but still remains under medical supervision. Brewer's yeast has helped alleviate the numbness in her hands and feet, and the healthy diet has led to a loss of several kilograms. Instead of feeling tired she now has more energy than before and plans to take up some gentle exercise such as swimming.

Do you need to lose weight?

It is vital to assess the reasons behind your motivation to start a weight-loss plan. Your primary considerations should be how you can improve your health and general well-being.

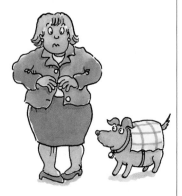

It's a tight fit!
Some people insist on squeezing into clothes that are clearly too small for them. Unfortunately this only serves to accentuate their curves.

Unfortunately many people adopt the wrong attitude to a weight-loss plan, often deciding to lose weight purely because they believe it will make them look more attractive. A more sensible approach is to recognise that your physical and psychological health is paramount and any weight-control plan should give priority to these considerations.

REASONS TO LOSE WEIGHT
For some, wanting to lose weight can be as simple as finding that favourite clothes no longer fit. This can be a valid reason, but you should also consider to what degree an increase in activity might help; for example, exercises that tone the stomach muscles may be all that is needed if the waistbands of your clothes have grown a little too tight.

Many people strongly associate being overweight with being unattractive and some see it as contributing to relationship problems, poor job prospects and reduced quality of life, and believe that weight loss will bring greater self-esteem. This focus on an improvement in appearance as the answer to life's problems is in many ways understandable. It is, after all, how the media encourage us to see the world. But the challenges and difficulties in life are far too complex to be resolved simply by a change in image and if this is the thinking behind a weight-loss programme, it may be doomed to failure from the start as the goal is too high to be realistically achieved.

It's important to think of weight control in terms of the health benefits associated with being within the recommended weight range for your age and height. Reducing the fat content of your diet and increasing activity are sensible, achievable steps to take that will help control weight and improve general health and well-being. For some people weight loss is essential for health reasons. If you are obese – if your BMI is over 30 (see page 25) – your health will benefit from even modest, but sustained, weight loss. For those with a BMI between 25 and 30, weight loss is advisable when other health risk factors are present: if you are a heavy smoker or drinker, for example, or if you suffer from hypertension or diabetes.

Health risks of being obese
The main cause of premature death among obese people is heart disease: hypertension, coronary thrombosis and congestive heart failure are all significantly more common among obese people than among those with a healthy weight. In fact, obesity in women

---

BURNING OFF CALORIES: *Swimming*

Swimming is an excellent cardio-respiratory exercise. It tones many problem areas of the body, and as it is non-weight-bearing it is ideal for pregnant women and people with joint or back pain.

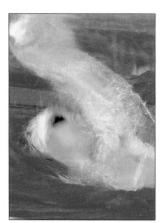

Muscle groups benefiting
Helps strengthen the back and abdominal muscles. Works the upper arms and pectoral muscles – breast stroke also works the thighs.

Equipment
Goggles will prevent eye irritation from chlorine.

Calories burnt
Twenty minutes of continuous swimming will burn about 170 calories.

is one of the best predictors of heart disease, after age and existing high blood pressure, as weight gain significantly increases some important risk factors for cardiovascular disease, specifically cholesterol, triglycerides, blood glucose and blood pressure.

Non-insulin-dependent diabetes mellitus (NIDDM) is a major cause of death in obese people. A man who is more than 40 per cent above his average weight is 5.2 times more likely to die of diabetes than a man of healthy weight; for women the ratio is 7.9 for a similar degree of excess weight.

Obese people are more likely to get gallstones, because their bile and excess adipose tissue (the body's connective tissue that stores fat) contains a lot of cholesterol.

Adipose tissue is a source of aromatase, the enzyme system that converts androgens (male sexual characteristic hormone) to oestrogens (female sexual characteristic hormone). Consequently, obese people have a higher circulating level of oestrogens compared with people of healthy weight. This probably explains why obese women have more menstrual problems, higher incidence of infertility, and irregular periods. It may also explain the increased prevalence of sex-hormone-sensitive cancers in obese women, such as malignant tumours of the breast, ovary, endometrium and cervix.

Psychological consequences

People who are overweight often suffer more from depression and low self-esteem than those of healthy weight. The strength of the stigma and distress associated with being overweight was illustrated by a study conducted in the United States in 1991 that looked at the morbid fear of weight regain in patients who had once been obese, but following surgery had lost weight and successfully maintained this weight loss for at least three years. In spite of the strong tendency for people to evaluate their own worst handicap as less disabling than other handicaps, patients said they would prefer to be an ideal weight with a major handicap (deaf, dyslexic, diabetic, legally blind, very bad acne, heart disease, or even one leg amputated) than to be extremely obese. All patients said they would rather be an ideal weight with the income they have now than an extremely obese multi-millionaire.

Feelings of embarrassment and self-hate about being overweight can lead to reduced physical activity and an increased feeling of isolation and insularity, which may cause a slide into depression.

Severely obese people can have difficulties in social situations because of their physical size. If they cannot fit into normal size chairs, they are virtually excluded from

PHYSICAL RISKS OF BEING OVERWEIGHT

In addition to increased risk of disease, being very overweight can also have harmful physical effects on your body.

▶ *Undue pressure placed on weight-bearing joints like hips and knees can result in osteoarthritis.*

▶ *Shortness of breath and general lethargy results from extra strain placed on the heart.*

▶ *Too much strain is placed on the back – backaches are common and existing back problems will be exacerbated.*

▶ *There is an increase in the risks associated with anaesthesia and surgery.*

WILL LOSING WEIGHT BENEFIT YOUR HEALTH?

Before you begin a weight-loss programme, you should consider the reasons behind your decision. The most important reason for choosing to lose weight is to benefit your health and well-being. If you are already overweight, factors such as smoking and the amount of exercise you take will make weight loss even more important. This quiz can help you determine if weight loss is appropriate for you. Score 4 each time you answer (a), 2 each time you answer (b) and 1 each time you answer (c). If none of the answers apply score 0. Whatever your score, improving your diet and taking more exercise will improve your fitness and body shape.

QUESTIONS	ANSWERS		
IS YOUR BMI (SEE PAGE 25):	(a) 30 or over	(b) Between 25 and 30	(c) Below 25
DO YOU HAVE ANY OF THE FOLLOWING MEDICAL PROBLEMS:	(a) High cholesterol, high blood pressure or diabetes	(b) Shortage of breath	(c) Indigestion or heartburn
DO YOU SMOKE CIGARETTES:	(a) Heavily – 20 or more a day	(b) Socially – 10 a day	(c) Seldom
IS YOUR WAIST-TO-HIP RATIO (SEE PAGE 24):	(a) 1.0 or above (man); 0.85 or above (woman)	(b) 9.5 or above (man); 0.75 or above (woman)	(c) Below 9.5 (man); below 0.75 (woman)
DO YOU EXERCISE FOR 20 MINUTES OR MORE:	(a) Seldom or never	(b) Once or twice a week	(c) More than twice a week
HOW DID YOU SCORE?	12–20: weight loss is advisable for health reasons	8–12: weight loss may improve your general health	Below 8: you probably do not need to lose weight

Waist-to-hip ratio

Your waist-to-hip ratio is a useful guide to whether the distribution of fat in your body is healthy. A waist-to-hip ratio above 1.0 in men; and above 0.85 in women is a signal of unhealthy fat distribution which can increase the risk of many diseases, including heart disease.

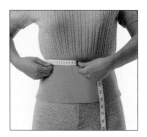

1 *Measure your waist – the point just above the top of your hip bones where your body naturally curves in.*

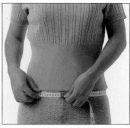

2 *Measure your hips at their widest point just above the buttocks. To calculate your waist-to-hip ratio divide your waist measurement by your hip measurement.*

attending social events such as the theatre or cinema, or even travelling by public transport unless they stand. These penalties all lead to an increase in the social isolation already felt by the obese person.

DECIDING TO LOSE WEIGHT

It is important to objectively assess the reasons why you want to lose weight. Your health is a very good reason for losing weight; if the health problem is sufficiently serious, many people find the motivation to reach a sensible weight and stay there.

Losing weight in order to feel more attractive, however, is a far more complicated issue. There may be a deeper emotional or psychological problem behind your desire to lose weight that needs looking at before a successful weight-control programme can be introduced. A recent study revealed that obesity can be a 'coat rack' where patients hang all their problems, failings and disturbing feelings. Some obese patients who have lost weight, subsequently found that the results and rewards they anticipated did not materialise and life's problems continued and even intensified.

Some people wrongly assume that they are a healthy weight when they need to accept that they are overweight and make a plan to rectify the situation. Correct assessment is essential. Do not guess your weight or height. Studies have shown that most men would like to think they are taller and more muscular than they really are, and most women would like to think that they are slimmer than they really are.

You will notice that there is no allowance for frame size in the BMI chart on page 25 – it is a myth that 'big bones' make a person heavier. People who are particularly muscular can be healthy at higher weights than people of average body composition; it is excess fat that is the problem, not excess muscle. Finally, being able to pinch an inch does not always mean that you are overweight; it tells you more about the state of your stomach muscles than about how much excess weight you have.

Your waist-to-hip ratio (see left) reveals if you carry more fat around your stomach and waist than on your thighs and bottom: a distribution which statistics have shown increases the possibilities of heart disease, high blood pressure, arthritis and non-insulin-dependent diabetes.

HOW DO YOU LOSE WEIGHT?

The key to weight loss is shifting the balance so that energy (calorie) intake is less than energy expenditure. When this happens, weight loss will occur. The way most people achieve this is to consume fewer calories and exercise more.

Exercise alone, with no change to your existing diet, may not help you to lose weight. For example, the body doesn't start to burn fat until you have been exercising for at least 20 minutes, and to lose 0.45 kg (1 lb) in weight through exercise you would need to perform 20 000 sit ups. However, even small amounts of exercise will assist in the burning of energy which means that your diet doesn't need to be unrealistically severe for you to start losing weight. Exercise will also increase the proportion of lean tissue to body fat which increases your metabolic rate. Dieting can in fact lower your metabolic rate so exercise will help balance this effect. Exercise will also improve your general health and will improve muscle tone and appearance.

In the same way, dieting without undertaking exercise may not lead to long-term weight loss. Exercise has been shown to be particularly important in maintaining a steady weight once the initial excess weight has been lost. Because regular exercise

WEIGHT MEASUREMENT

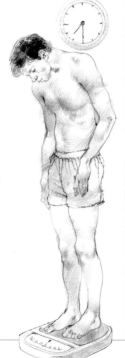

Always weigh yourself first thing in the morning, after going to the lavatory. Use the same set of scales throughout your weight-control programme as scales can vary widely, even those in GP surgeries and hospitals.

GETTING IT RIGHT Make sure your scales are accurate and placed on a hard, level surface.

THE BODY MASS INDEX

Your Body Mass Index is a good way to check your weight is healthy. Calculate it from this chart by locating your weight at the side of the table and lining it up with your height. Being overweight is defined as having a BMI greater than 25. If you have a BMI of over 30, your health could be at risk and you should see your doctor.

WEIGHT (kg)	HEIGHT (cm)																
	150	152.5	155	157.5	160	162.5	165	167.5	170	172.5	175	177.5	180	182.5	185	187.5	190
40	18	17	17	16	16	15	15	14	14	13	13	13	12	12	12	11	11
41	18	18	17	17	16	16	15	15	14	14	13	13	13	12	12	12	11
42	19	18	17	17	16	16	15	15	15	14	14	13	13	13	12	12	12
43	19	18	18	17	17	16	16	15	15	14	14	14	13	13	13	12	12
44	20	19	18	18	17	17	16	16	15	15	15	14	14	13	13	13	12
45	20	19	19	18	18	17	17	16	16	15	15	15	14	14	13	13	12
46	20	20	19	19	18	17	17	16	16	15	15	15	14	14	13	13	13
47	21	20	20	19	18	18	17	17	16	16	15	15	15	14	14	13	13
48	21	21	20	19	19	18	18	17	17	16	16	15	15	14	14	14	13
49	22	21	20	20	19	19	18	17	17	16	16	16	15	15	14	14	14
50	22	21	21	20	20	19	18	18	17	17	16	16	15	15	15	14	14
51	23	22	21	21	20	19	19	18	18	17	17	16	16	15	15	15	14
52	23	22	21	20	20	20	19	19	18	17	17	17	16	16	15	15	14
53	24	23	22	21	21	20	19	19	18	18	17	17	16	16	15	15	15
54	24	23	22	22	21	20	20	19	19	18	18	17	17	17	16	16	15
55	24	24	23	22	21	21	20	20	19	18	18	17	17	17	16	16	15
56	25	24	23	23	22	21	21	20	19	19	18	18	17	17	16	16	16
57	25	25	24	23	22	22	21	20	20	19	19	18	18	17	17	16	16
58	26	25	24	23	23	22	21	21	20	19	19	18	18	17	17	16	16
59	26	25	25	24	23	22	22	21	20	20	19	19	18	18	17	17	16
60	27	26	25	24	23	23	22	21	21	20	20	19	19	18	18	17	17
61	27	26	25	25	24	23	22	22	21	20	20	19	19	18	18	17	17
62	28	27	26	25	24	23	23	22	21	21	20	20	19	19	18	18	17
63	28	27	26	25	25	24	23	22	22	21	21	20	19	19	18	18	17
64	28	28	27	26	25	24	24	23	22	22	21	20	20	19	19	18	18
65	29	28	27	26	25	25	24	23	22	22	21	21	20	20	19	18	18
66	29	28	27	27	26	25	24	24	23	22	22	21	20	20	19	19	18
67	30	29	28	27	26	25	25	24	23	23	22	21	21	20	20	19	19
68	30	29	28	27	27	26	25	24	24	23	22	22	21	20	20	19	19
69	31	30	29	28	27	26	25	25	24	23	23	22	21	21	20	20	19
70	31	30	29	28	27	27	26	25	24	24	23	22	22	21	20	20	19
71	32	31	30	29	28	27	26	25	25	24	23	23	22	21	21	20	20
72	32	31	30	29	28	27	26	26	25	24	24	23	22	22	21	20	20
73	32	31	30	29	29	28	27	26	25	25	24	23	23	22	21	21	20
74	33	32	31	30	29	28	27	26	26	25	24	23	23	22	22	21	20
75	33	32	31	30	29	28	28	27	26	25	24	24	23	23	22	21	21
76	34	33	32	31	30	29	28	27	26	25	24	24	23	23	22	22	21
77	34	33	32	31	30	29	28	27	27	26	25	24	24	23	23	22	21
78	35	34	32	31	30	30	29	28	27	26	25	25	24	23	23	22	22
79	35	34	33	32	31	30	29	28	27	27	26	25	24	24	23	22	22
80	36	34	33	32	31	30	29	29	28	27	26	25	25	24	23	23	22
81	36	35	34	33	32	31	30	29	28	27	26	26	25	24	24	23	22
82	36	35	34	33	32	31	30	29	28	28	27	26	25	25	24	23	23
83	37	36	35	33	32	31	30	30	29	28	27	26	26	25	24	24	23
84	37	36	35	34	33	32	31	30	29	28	27	27	26	25	25	24	23
85	38	37	35	34	33	34	31	30	29	29	28	27	26	26	25	24	24
86	38	37	36	35	34	33	32	31	30	29	29	28	27	26	25	25	24
87	39	37	36	35	34	33	32	31	30	29	28	28	27	26	25	25	24
88	39	38	37	35	34	33	32	31	30	30	29	28	27	26	26	25	24
89	40	38	37	36	35	34	33	32	31	30	29	28	27	27	26	25	25
90	40	39	37	36	35	34	33	32	31	30	29	29	28	27	26	26	25
91	40	39	38	37	36	34	33	32	31	31	30	29	28	27	27	26	25
92	41	40	38	37	36	35	34	33	32	31	30	29	28	28	27	26	25
93	41	40	39	37	36	35	34	33	32	31	30	30	29	28	27	26	26
94	42	40	39	38	37	36	35	34	33	32	31	30	29	28	27	27	26
95	42	41	40	38	37	36	35	34	33	32	31	30	29	29	28	27	26
96	43	41	40	39	38	36	35	34	33	32	31	30	30	29	28	27	27
97	43	42	40	39	38	37	36	35	34	33	32	31	30	29	28	28	27
98	44	42	41	40	38	37	36	35	34	33	32	31	30	29	29	28	27
99	44	43	41	40	39	37	36	35	34	33	32	31	31	30	29	28	27
100	44	43	42	40	39	38	37	36	35	34	33	32	31	30	29	28	28

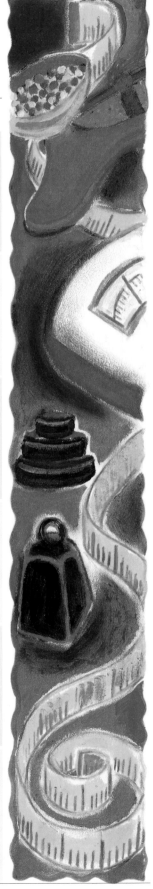

How much weight should you expect to lose each week?

Losing weight is a slow process. If you consume 1000 calories per day less than you expend, then you should lose between 0.5 kg to 1 kg (1 to 2 lb) per week. This represents a healthy and sustainable weight loss. Don't be discouraged if your weight loss is no greater than this. Many people give up on a diet because in their view it is not working, but losing a large amount of weight fast can have health risks and is harder to sustain.

burns off extra energy you will be able to eat a more 'normal' diet without drastic eating restrictions.

Therapies and surgical intervention

For some seriously obese people, a more drastic approach is sometimes prescribed for weight loss. There are many types of drugs for the treatment of obesity, but these do have potential drawbacks. In the short term, appetite suppressants (or anorectic drugs) help weight loss, but patients often regain weight when they stop taking the drugs. Some patients ask for a drug to speed up their metabolic rate. Large doses of thyroid hormone have been shown to do just this, but unfortunately the resulting weight loss is mainly lean tissue, not fat. Other drugs which increase metabolic rate have more dangerous consequences including increased risk of heart problems.

Surgical procedures include gastric stapling, or a gastric bypass. In gastric stapling a line of staples is punched through the stomach so that only about 50 ml (2 fl oz) of food can be taken at any one time. A gastric bypass is an operation in which the gut is cut and rejoined to provide a relatively short exposure of the food to the action of digestive enzymes, while the majority of the bowel is short-circuited. This means that less food is actually absorbed by the body. Weight loss is usually rapid following these operations, but unfortunately these procedures are not without risks – there have been a number of deaths and all patients undergoing such operations need ongoing medical supervision.

One of the more successful treatments for weight control is behavioural therapy. The idea behind behavioural therapy for obesity is that eating behaviour is learned, and that obese people have learnt a type of eating behaviour which leads to weight gain. Behavioural therapy helps the person learn new eating patterns. For example, for the overweight patient who binge eats, the key to success is to identify what triggers these binges, and work from there, either by avoiding the triggers or learning how to deal with them in a way which doesn't involve eating. As with all weight management programmes, behavioural therapy is most successful when it is combined with lifelong changes to eating habits and a permanent increase in physical activity.

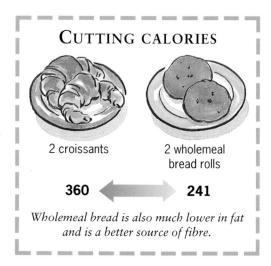

CUTTING CALORIES

2 croissants   2 wholemeal bread rolls

360 ⬅➡ 241

Wholemeal bread is also much lower in fat and is a better source of fibre.

Diet and weight control for everyone

For anyone embarking on a diet and exercise programme, the aim should be weight control rather than dramatic weight loss in the short term. People who are constantly on diets (yo-yo dieters), and whose weight fluctuates over time, are less likely to report good physical health and often express a significantly lower sense of general well-being, worse mental health and greater stress than those who maintain their weight. Furthermore, there is some evidence that yo-yo dieting may make the obese patient more vulnerable to binge behaviour. Maintaining a stable weight after weight loss should be seen as just as important as the initial loss of weight. It is much better to lose a little weight and keep it off, than to lose a significant amount only to regain it.

Set yourself a realistic target weight, but also set a number of interim targets. The goal is often so far away from the starting point that without small victories along the way you may be tempted to give up as you realise the long and difficult task before you.

The key to successful long-term weight loss is to make small but significant and permanent changes to your diet and activity level. Start a food diary so that you can easily assess if your diet follows recommended guidelines delivering all the nutrients your body needs in the correct proportions (see page 51). Look at ways of reducing the fat in your diet such as substituting low-fat alternatives for high-fat dairy products and grilling instead of frying. Try to improve your fitness level by gradually increasing the amount of exercise you do each week (see Chapter 5) until you exercise for at least 20 minutes or more, five times a week.

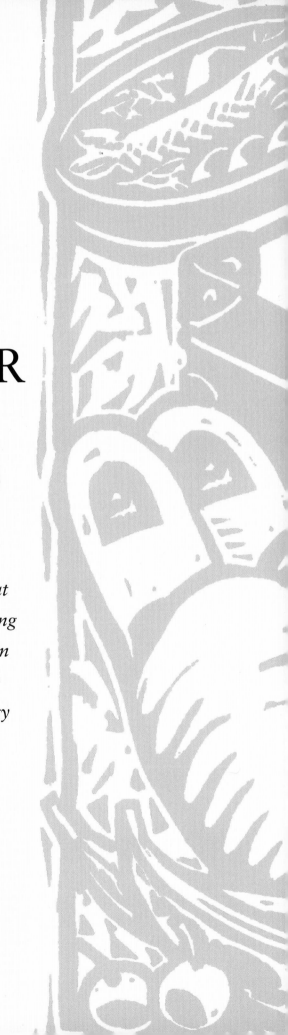

CHAPTER 2

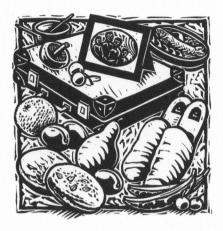

WHY IS YOUR BODY THE SHAPE IT IS?

Weight is influenced by a number of factors that interact in complex ways. The primary controlling factor is the energy content of the food we eat in relation to our energy requirements, but other factors such as metabolism, genetics, psychology and the environment all play important roles.

THE PHYSIOLOGY OF WEIGHT CONTROL

Weight is affected by the interaction of a number of physiological factors including appetite, metabolism, hormones and heredity, most of which can be influenced by your actions.

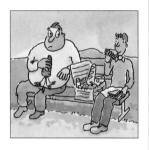

CAUSE AND EFFECT
Regular exercise gives a higher energy expenditure than a sedentary lifestyle and will burn off extra calories instead of storing them as fat. This means the calorie intake of an active person can be higher than that of someone who is inactive.

There are many physiological reasons that have contributed to making you the weight you now are. Some, such as your genetic make-up, you have no control over. But there are other areas, such as the body's metabolism, where you can implement change for the better.

HUNGER AND APPETITE

It is important to understand the difference between hunger and appetite in order to help control the factors that make you want to eat. Hunger is a direct physiological message sent by your body to alert you to the fact that food is required for your survival. It occurs when the stomach is empty and blood sugar levels are running low. Appetite, on the other hand, is a desire for and anticipation of food that may not reflect a physical need for it. Even before food enters the mouth, the sight and smell causes the stomach and intestines to prepare for food. Appetite can override the fact that hunger has been satisfied and so has an important role in the amount of energy taken into the body through food and drink. Endorphin, the body's natural painkiller and mood elevator, may also play a part in appetite. Studies show that higher levels of endorphins are released in obese people after they have eaten. This may explain why obese people appear to be 'addicted' to food.

How the body senses satiety

The body's regulatory mechanisms are self-programmed to ensure that it gets enough energy (calories) by initiating the drive to eat whenever it has an under supply of energy.

HOW THE BRAIN CONTROLS APPETITE

Appetite is regulated by a part of the brain called the hypothalamus that monitors 'appetite factors', such as the levels of nutrients (e.g. glucose) and other chemicals in the blood. It also gets signals from 'stretch sensors' in the stomach which indicate if it is empty or full. The hypothalamus then stimulates the drive to eat when necessary. Following a meal these 'appetite factors' subside and the hypothalamus sends out 'satiety' signals which suppress the appetite. But these signals are slower to work which can lead to overeating.

Hypothalamus monitors the status of 'appetite factors' and gut 'stretch sensors' and activates or suppresses appetite

Salivary glands release saliva containing digestive enzymes to begin food breakdown

Liver stores excess sugar following a meal and slowly releases it as needed by the body

BRAIN CONTROL
Appetite involves a complex system that is regulated by a tiny region of the brain.

Olfactory (smell) organ and taste buds detect presence of food and activate salivary glands and digestive enzyme-producing cells in stomach

Stomach releases digestive enzymes to continue food breakdown. Stretch receptors indicate when stomach is full

Small intestine detects food leaving stomach and produces digestive enzymes to continue food breakdown. Absorbs nutrients into bloodstream

But the opposing mechanism to stop eating when enough energy has been consumed, does not appear to operate quite so effectively; overeating does not produce powerful signals to cut down. Numerous studies have demonstrated that if we have access to an abundant supply of palatable, high-fat food we tend to overeat. This is often called 'passive over-consumption', which means that we continue to eat the same amount of food, but the calorie intake is much higher because fat is more energy dense than carbohydrate or protein.

The body's weak defences against overeating means that most people find it easy to do. Undereating, however, requires more effort and will-power and is a deliberate act.

METABOLISM

The process by which food is broken down to release energy is known as metabolism. The energy is used to perform various functions, such as keeping the heart beating, maintaining liver function and providing fuel for exercise and physical activity.

If your weight is stable then the amount of energy (measured in calories or joules) you are eating is equal to the amount you use. If you eat too much it is stored as fat. To lose weight you must eat fewer calories than you burn off.

How much energy your body uses depends on a number of factors. The main determinant is the Basal Metabolic Rate (BMR). This is the amount of energy used by the body for functions such as breathing or making your heart beat and producing heat. In other words it is the amount of energy needed to keep you ticking over. This is influenced by age, gender, body size, nutritional and physical status as well as genetics. You also use up additional energy during physical activity and exercise.

What affects metabolism

The amount of exercise you do is the main influence on the body's metabolic rate. The more active you are the faster your metabolism will be, increasing the energy that you burn. In time, with regular exercise, it is possible to increase your resting metabolic rate so that your body uses more energy for every action from breathing to sport.

There are also a number of substances that can cause a change in the amount of energy the body uses. Nicotine and caffeine cause small but measurable increases in the metabolic rate. Agents such as amphetamines, thyroxine and some drugs used in the treatment of obesity also cause an increase.

Illness and disease can also increase the body's metabolic rate. For example, in Graves disease the thyroid gland is overactive, making the body use more energy than normal. The metabolic rate also increases in response to stress and fear.

Other drugs reduce energy expenditure, such as beta-blockers, drugs used in the treatment of angina and hypertension, for the prevention of migraine and to control an overactive thyroid gland. They may also produce slight weight gain.

Raising your metabolism

Exercise will increase your metabolic rate but to make significant changes that alter your body composition you need to exercise on a regular basis – not one post-Christmas exercise session that leads to aching muscles and can put a sudden strain on the heart. Regular moderate exercise for 20–30 minutes a day is more beneficial than intensive one hour sessions once or twice a week.

It is important to fit exercise into your day-to-day life and to find a form of exercise that you enjoy so that carrying it out is not a boring task. There are many simple ways of introducing more regular activity into your life. Ask yourself do you need to get a bus for only two stops? Do you need to take the lift up two floors? Could you go out for a walk at lunch time?

There are no foods that will burn off fat; it is a misconception that grapefruit or other foods will melt fat away or boost your metabolism. Also without scientific foundation are claims that a special mixture of foods taken in a certain way will have a magical effect, or a particular nutrient mix will increase your energy output. Such diets only work if they help you to restrict your total energy intake.

Unfortunately dieting itself will lower your metabolic rate, rather than raise it. When your intake of food drops, your metabolic rate slows down to enable you to function using as little energy and stored fat as possible. This is

continued on page 32

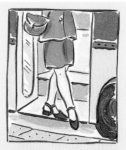

QUICK FITNESS TIP
Get off the bus two stops before you normally do and walk the rest of the way.

HIGH ENERGY NEEDS
After years of following strenuous training regimes athletes develop such a high metabolic rate that they must consume large quantities of food every day just to keep pace with their energy needs.

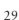

Metabolism

Including some activity in your working day will boost your metabolism, which can otherwise slow down if you are inactive, especially if you are also on a diet. There are positive steps you can take from the moment you wake up to the end of the day.

To boost your metabolism, exercise is needed in your day-to-day life. If you work in an office, you probably sit behind a desk or computer screen all day. You may feel sluggish or lethargic on waking or feel that you cannot function without constant caffeine boosts. But the best pick-me-up at any time of the day is some gentle exercise. The exercises shown here can be practised anywhere and at any time, without the need for a lot of space, expensive equipment, or too much spare time.

At first, you may find it difficult to stretch as far as you feel you should but don't worry, it is important not to push your muscles too far and to stop if you feel any pain. With daily perseverance you will quickly notice a marked improvement in your suppleness and energy levels, as well as in your mental agility.

It may be a good deal easier for you to adopt an exercise routine successfully if you get the support of your work colleagues. Try and get them to join in as much as possible.

7 am As soon as you get out of bed perform some simple stretches, such as the two on this page, to start your blood flowing and warm up joints and muscles. Try to hold each stretch for 8-10 seconds but relax slowly if you begin to feel tense or sore.

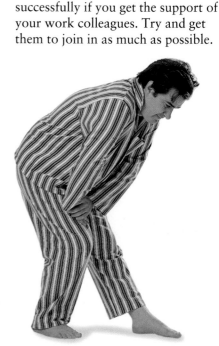

OVERHEAD STRETCH
Stand with your feet hip width apart, your back straight and your head in line with your spine. Lift your arms above your head and reach as far upwards as you can with your palms touching. To extend the stretch further, ease your arms back slightly. Repeat five times.

HAMSTRING STRETCH
Stand with your feet apart. Keeping your chest lifted and your stomach pulled in, take a step forward with your left leg, keeping it straight. Bend your right knee and lean forward from the hips, lowering your chest toward your right thigh. Hold the stretch. Repeat with the other leg.

8 am Find a more energetic way to get to work. Try to avoid driving your car if possible. Can you walk to a railway station? If you catch a bus, can you walk briskly for 20 minutes to a bus stop further from your home? Do some gentle

stretches as you walk – swing your arms and flex your fingers by opening and closing your hand as a fist. You can also use this time to become aware of how your body feels as it moves and which movements work which muscles.

9 am At the office, use the stairs rather than the lift to get to your floor and keep using the stairs throughout the day if you have to run errands between floors. Try to pace your climb so you are not exhausted at the end of it.

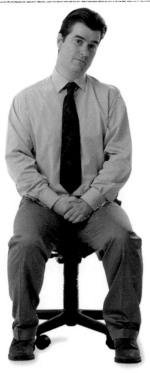

11 **am** Don't be tempted to have a biscuit or cake for your mid-morning break. Instead try to persuade your colleagues to join you in a series of stretches. This is particularly important if you sit in front of a computer terminal most of the day as muscles can become stiff if you remain in one position for long periods of time.

NECK STRETCH

Sitting with your back straight and your chest lifted, clasp your hands loosely in front of you and relax your shoulders. Keeping your shoulders still, slowly incline your left ear towards your left shoulder. When you have tilted your head as far as is comfortable, hold the stretch. Repeat the exercise to the right.

ARM STRETCH

Clasp your hands behind your back and slowly lift your arms up, keeping your elbows straight. Hold for a few seconds.

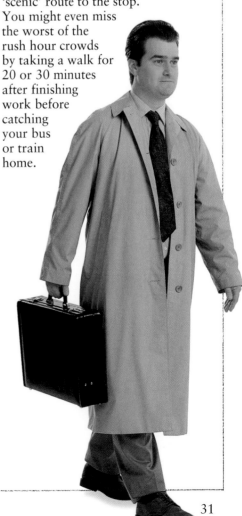

1 **pm** In the second half of your lunch hour take time out for a brisk walk around the local streets. The change of scene will also serve to restore your concentration.

3 **pm** Mid-afternoon, perform some more stretches – choose ones which target different muscles from those worked on earlier. There are plenty that can be done at your desk.

6 **pm** If your usual railway station or bus stop is close to your office try to walk to a station or stop a little farther away; or take a 'scenic' route to the stop. You might even miss the worst of the rush hour crowds by taking a walk for 20 or 30 minutes after finishing work before catching your bus or train home.

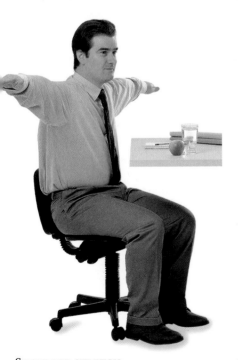

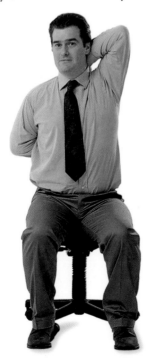

SHOULDER STRETCH

Keeping your arms level with your shoulders, extend them away from your body and reach out as far as is comfortable. Make small circles by rotating your arms backwards five times and then forwards five times.

TRICEP STRETCH

Place your left hand behind your back so that your palm sits between your shoulder blades and your elbow points upwards. Bring your right hand up behind your back and try to join hands. Hold, then repeat with the other arm.

the body's in-built protection mechanism against starvation. After being on a diet for two weeks, your metabolic rate can drop by as much as 10 per cent. Exercise can help to prevent this fall, so it is crucial for successful weight loss. Dieting on its own will mean the body simply becomes more efficient at functioning on less food.

Changes in metabolism over time

Your metabolism can change during your lifetime because of a number of factors. There is a small decrease in BMR with age – about 1–2 per cent up to the age of 60 and slightly more after this. But a much more significant contributor to a lower BMR is the widespread decrease in physical activity that usually occurs as people get older. If you are not as active as you once were, then the amount of muscle in your body dwindles and you don't need as much energy. The weight gain often associated with ageing is possibly because diet has not changed even though energy expenditure is reduced.

THE LIPOSTAT THEORY

There is a theory that the amount of fat in the body governs appetite and energy intake. The cornerstone to this theory is that the body has a preset genetically determined body fat mass. The sensors for this are in the brain, in particular, the hypothalamus and in and around the appetite control centres. An unknown chemical released from the adipose tissue signals to the hypothalamus the state of the body's energy stores. To put it simply, it works like a central heating system. The hypothalamus is the thermostat and sensors are found in fat tissue. Depending on the state of the fat stores, it drives or suppresses appetite in an attempt to maintain their level. However, like any other thermostat it is not perfect and small fluctuations in intake cannot be sensed. One theory is that even very few calories above your required daily intake can lead to a large weight gain in the long term. This cannot be picked up by the thermostat initially, and the difference may be so slight that the thermostat resets itself. But when you want to lose weight and decrease your calorie intake substantially, the thermostat interprets the drop as a starvation warning and sends powerful signals that you are hungry.

HORMONES

Many hormones are involved in appetite control and the number that have been identified grows constantly. Insulin is known to have an effect on appetite and weight, and thyroid hormones and sex hormones also play an important part.

The role of insulin

Two hormones produced by the pancreas control blood sugar levels in the body. Glucagon stimulates the breakdown of carbohydrate stored in the liver and muscles into glucose or sugar which is then released into the bloodstream. Insulin lowers blood sugar levels by stimulating the uptake of glucose by the body's cells. The theory that insulin and other hormones from the pancreas have a role in feeding behaviour is not new, but remains controversial.

Injection of a small amount of insulin produces a slight fall in blood glucose levels and this can trigger the urge to eat. This is probably because the hypothalamus detects the lower levels of glucose in the blood and initiates the desire to eat to make up the deficit. It is also possible that insulin plays a part in the satiety response. After eating, insulin levels drop in the brain as well as in the body tissues and this may play a part in inhibiting the desire to eat.

DISTRIBUTION OF FAT IN MEN AND WOMEN

The sex hormones that control fat distribution (see page 34) are different in men and women resulting in different body shapes. Added to this is the fact that most women carry about 10 per cent more fat than men of similar build.

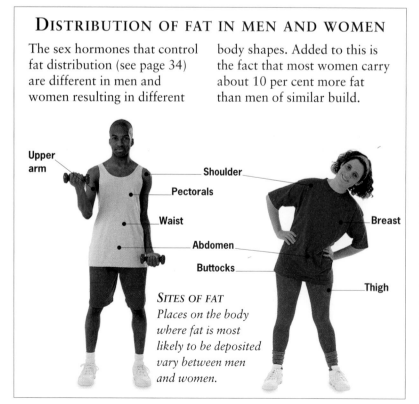

Upper arm

Shoulder

Pectorals

Waist

Breast

Abdomen

Buttocks

Thigh

SITES OF FAT
Places on the body where fat is most likely to be deposited vary between men and women.

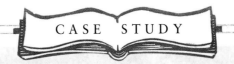
The Overweight Family

If all the members of a family are overweight this may indicate that there is a genetic predisposition to weight gain. But your genetic make-up doesn't have to dictate your weight. Changes in diet and exercise can result in major improvements in health, fitness and weight that will overcome the genetic influences and enable individuals to consciously control their body shape.

Susan, 46, has recently returned to work after being a housewife and mother for 13 years. She has begun to feel self-conscious about her weight – she gained 19 kg (3 stone) over the past ten years. Her husband has also mentioned that he feels uncomfortable about his weight. Susan knows that the children don't enjoy sport at school and realises that they may be unhappy because of their weight too. Susan has tried dieting before but has always put the weight back on. This time she has decided to make long-term changes in the lifestyle and eating habits of the whole family that will benefit them all. After talking to her doctor and doing some reading for ideas, Susan called a family conference.

WHAT SHOULD THE FAMILY DO?

Susan needs to reduce the amount of fried foods that she prepares for the family and use other cooking methods such as grilling and baking. She should also substitute fish, poultry or a vegetarian meal for their usual red meat on three to four nights a week. The family needs to control their habitual snacking in the evenings: instead of watching television they should find family-orientated activities such as playing outdoor games, going swimming or even playing boardgames that will distract them from the urge to snack. As the family doesn't do any physical exercise, they should start introducing joint activities such as walks or cycle rides that can be fun for both adults and children.

Action Plan

EATING HABITS
Gradually decrease the amount of fat and sugar-laden foods from the family's meals and reduce evening snacking. Use fruit and vegetables as healthy snacks and substitute fruit for high-calorie desserts.

DIET
Roast, grill or poach skinless chicken. Bake potatoes in their jackets. Trim visible fat from meat and cut down on fried foods.

EXERCISE
Walk to and from school with the children to burn calories. Find an activity the whole family enjoys and make it a weekly event.

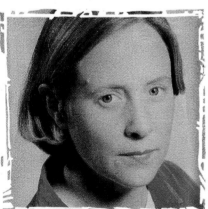

EXERCISE
Lack of exercise means little fat is burned as energy.

EATING HABITS
A diet that is high in fatty foods will not always satisfy hunger and can lead to the urge to reach for snacks, which are also usually high in fat.

DIET
Untrimmed meat increases the fat content of a meal significantly. Cooking foods in fat adds extra calories.

HOW THINGS TURNED OUT FOR THE FAMILY

Susan took time to plan the family meals around healthy eating principles and shopped accordingly. Instead of buying treats, she made sure that there was always fruit in the house for snacks. An evening cookery course gave her new meal ideas. The family began swimming together regularly and as they lost weight the children started to show more interest in school sports. After three months Susan lost 10 kg (1.5 stone) and her confidence at work began to increase.

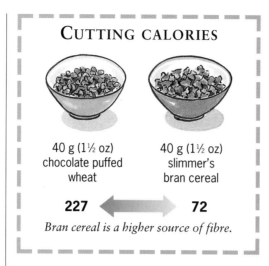

CUTTING CALORIES

40 g (1½ oz) chocolate puffed wheat

40 g (1½ oz) slimmer's bran cereal

227 ⟷ **72**

Bran cereal is a higher source of fibre.

Thyroid hormones

Thyroid hormones regulate the body's metabolism. Disorders that cause insufficient thyroid production, or hypothyroidism, can cause the body to put on weight, while overproduction of thyroid hormones, known as hyperthyroidism, can cause weight loss. Synthetic thyroid hormone drugs are used to treat both problems.

Although there have been some studies conducted on using thyroid hormones to help obese people lose weight, the numerous side effects and excessive loss of lean tissue rather than fat, have meant such treatments have not been successful.

Sex hormones

The male and female sex hormones control fat distribution. The male hormone testosterone concentrates fat around the stomach. Testosterone also appears to lead to an increase in appetite in people who take the hormone. The female sex hormone, oestrogen, concentrates fat distribution around the buttocks and thighs. Oestrogen and fat are also strongly linked in that a certain amount of fat is necessary to enable the body to produce sufficient levels of oestrogen. This is part of nature's way of ensuring that women have sufficient energy levels for reproduction.

Oestrogen-containing pills, such as oral contraceptives, can lead to weight gain in some women, but why this occurs is not clear. As the pill increases the level of oestrogen in the body it is thought that it further accentuates a woman's natural tendency to store excess fat and it may also stimulate appetite.

Many women report weight gain after menopause. Again, exactly why this should be the case is not clear. What is known is that a woman's fat distribution changes at this time due to a drop in oestrogen levels, and that she is more likely to start putting on weight around the stomach rather than the bottom and thighs (see page 19).

THE THYROID GLAND AND WEIGHT

An underactive or overactive thyroid gland can lead to some weight problems, however it is a misconception that these conditions are common. In fact, thyroid problems only affect about 1 per cent of the adult population. Situated at the front of the neck, the thyroid is one of the main hormone glands helping to regulate the body's energy levels. Correct production of thyroid hormones is crucial for promoting normal physical growth and mental development in children and for controlling your metabolic rate.

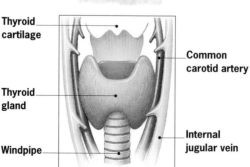

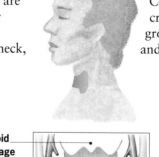

Thyroid cartilage

Common carotid artery

Thyroid gland

Internal jugular vein

Windpipe

HYPERTHYROIDISM
The overproduction of hormones by the thyroid gland causes symptoms such as fatigue, anxiety, sweating, intolerance to heat, diarrhoea, palpitations and weight loss. Treatment may involve part-removal of the gland, taking drugs to inhibit hormone production or, especially in older people, a dose of radioactive iodine to destroy some of the thyroid tissue.

HYPOTHYROIDISM
An underactive thyroid leads to insufficient thyroid hormone production, causing symptoms such as tiredness, dry skin, hair loss, sensitivity to cold, constipation and weight gain. Treatment is usually in the form of prescribed doses of the thyroid hormone thyroxin and this generally has to be continued for the rest of the sufferer's life.

HEREDITY

There is little doubt that heredity has a role to play in determining weight, but how large a part is still being debated. There is considerable evidence for a genetic predisposition to obesity. Identical twins are twice as likely to have a similar height-to-weight ratio, or Body Mass Index (BMI), than are non-identical twins. Studies show a relationship between the BMI of adult adoptees and their biological parents, but there is no correlation with their adoptive parents.

Genetic factors

Recently there has been much excitement about the discovery of a genetic fault in some mice that causes obesity. The genetic fault means that the mice do not produce enough of a protein called leptin which appears to help control weight. A similar gene has been identified in humans but the theory is complicated by the fact that obese people have more leptin in their blood than thin people. This suggests that in humans the leptin being produced is not working effectively, whereas in obese mice insufficient leptin is produced.

This protein could be the previously unknown factor released from fat identified in the Lipostat Theory (see page 32).

Although human trials of leptin have already begun, even if they are successful, it will be many years before this leads to a new treatment for obesity.

Moreover, there is probably no single gene that causes obesity in humans. Rather, a combination of genes is involved which makes identification much more difficult and makes it unlikely that any one treatment will help everyone.

Foetal nourishment

One of the discoveries made recently is that the nourishment a foetus receives may affect that person's health in later life. Professor David Barker and his team in Southampton in the early 1990s studied birth records, such as birth weight and length, of a group of people born in Herefordshire from 1911 onwards. They were able to trace these people as adults and record their state of health, or discover their cause of death. The results showed that babies who are born at full term, but are lighter than expected, have more health problems later on in life. One theory for this is that the mother's poor diet

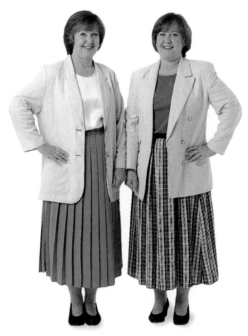

NATURE AND NURTURE
Identical twins are often the same weight and build when adults, even if raised by different parents. This shows the important part genes play in development.

may cause a decrease in the number of cells formed in the pancreas, thus putting the baby at risk later of diabetes. The baby may also adapt to its poor diet by becoming very efficient at storing nutrients, and later in life this may lead to a greater risk of diabetes and heart disease. An increased risk of obesity might also result, although this has not yet been shown

Not all studies, however, show the same effect. There is probably an interplay between genetic susceptibility to disease, the baby's environment in the womb and other events later in life that together determine the likelihood of chronic illnesses.

BURNING OFF CALORIES: *Cycling*

Cycling is a good all-over aerobic activity that can be used to develop cardiovascular fitness. As a low-impact exercise it can be a helpful activity for people with joint problems.

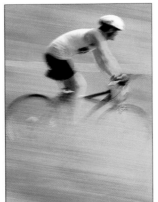

MUSCLE GROUPS BENEFITING
All of the leg muscles will benefit including the quadriceps (thigh muscle) and the gastrocnemius (calf muscle).

EQUIPMENT
A roadworthy bicycle and a bicycle helmet, or an indoor exercise bike.

CALORIES BURNT
At 16 km (10 miles) per hour, you expend 9 calories per minute: that's 540 calories per hour.

PSYCHOLOGICAL FACTORS

Your emotional state and the way you perceive yourself can have a direct influence on your weight; for many people it is often the determining factor in their weight problem.

Psychological factors play a major role in influencing your eating habits. Most people are aware that extreme psychological factors are involved in the dieting disorders anorexia nervosa and bulimia nervosa; but emotional problems and perceptions can also affect our everyday eating habits and weight in a variety of ways.

Research focusing on eating disorders has revealed just how close the relationship is between your psychological state and eating impulses. Anxiety, stress and depression can lead both to appetite loss and to the opposite – food cravings and binge eating. The foods most commonly craved are those that are sugar-laden and high in fat; research indicates that these foods may increase mood-elevating chemicals in the brain.

Studies carried out from 1989 to 1991 by Dr Ulrike Schmidt of the Institute of Psychiatry in London have shown that there is a clear link between anxiety and stress and the development of anorexia and bulimia. Her studies also showed that major life events, such as a death in the family or a divorce, precipitated onset of eating disorders

STEPS TOWARDS A BETTER SELF-IMAGE

It is easy to become too focused on a desire to lose weight. You can quickly become too scathing of yourself leading to a lack of self-confidence and depression. If a weight-loss programme is to be successful it must be fuelled with conviction and this requires a healthy self-image and the right motivation. Here are some suggestions on how to boost your self-esteem.

▶ *Read fashion magazines that portray glamorous models with a more critical eye. It is important to recognise that these images are highly stylised – professional make-up, lighting and camera angles are used to manufacture the perfect images we see in magazines and on television.*
▶ *Assess what is truly important in your life. Making a list of priorities in terms of career, travel, study, or relationship commitments can put body image into perspective.*
▶ *Turn your attention towards something other than your weight. Weight loss is a long-term commitment; for a short-term confidence boost try a new hair style, or have a make-up lesson.*
▶ *Stop thinking negatively. If you think of something negative, write it down then think of a positive statement to counteract it.*
▶ *Take time to look through your wardrobe and choose outfits that you feel good in. Opt for flattering styles that skim over problem areas like stomach and hips. Long-line jackets and blouses and long flowing skirts have a slimming effect.*

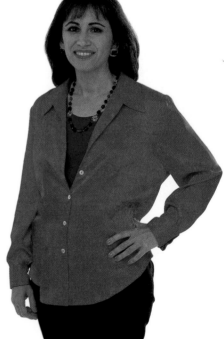

COLOUR WITH CONFIDENCE
Being bold with colours and jewellery to create a style which makes you feel confident will help detract attention from your weight.

A Bulimia Sufferer

Between 2 and 4 per cent of women are thought to have bulimia nervosa. Most of them keep it a secret. Although occasional overeating is perfectly normal, for example in a social setting, the kind of loss of control over their eating habits that women with bulimia nervosa experience can be both very distressing and harmful to their well-being if kept up for a prolonged period of time.

Alice is 32 and lives on her own. She developed bulimia nervosa after divorcing her husband two years ago. Since her divorce she has suffered bouts of depression and has begun to feel increasingly lonely and isolated. Pressure at work has meant she has had to take on more tasks than she can cope with. As a result she has been working very late and spending most evenings alone in her flat. Although she used to be very active, since her work load increased she has not had time to go to the gym at night and has started missing meals to try to lose weight. The stress of work and her loneliness at home has led Alice to binge, and the guilt and disgust she feels towards herself forces her to vomit afterwards.

WHAT SHOULD ALICE DO?

Alice needs to come to terms with the divorce from her husband and her other emotional needs and consulting a counsellor may help. She needs to recognise the link between her emotional health and her eating patterns.

She should also take steps to alleviate her sense of isolation at home. Setting aside time for doing things she enjoys, like going out with friends or seeing a film, is especially important whenever Alice feels like bingeing. Exercise may help boost her mood and relieve stress so making time for gym sessions may also help. Learning to say 'no' politely to her supervisor is another important first step.

Action Plan

STRESS
Learn to relax: take a bath, listen to music, or become involved in an interesting pastime to alleviate stress.

EMOTIONAL HEALTH
Organise a meeting with a counsellor to discuss and help overcome underlying emotions.

EATING HABITS
Regulate eating habits by eating three balanced meals a day. Eat healthy snacks such as fruit between meals to help control weight.

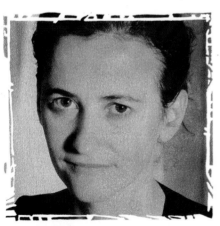

STRESS
Strain and stress often seem to play a role in bulimia nervosa. Developing effective ways of coping can reduce stress.

EATING HABITS
Missing meals to lose weight makes people more hungry, which makes overeating more likely later in the day.

EMOTIONAL HEALTH
Emotional problems such as grief and depression are often associated with eating disorders.

HOW THINGS TURNED OUT FOR ALICE

Alice negotiated a fairer distribution of the work load and left earlier at night. She felt less tired, started enjoying her free time again and began seeing a counsellor, who made her feel more positive about herself after showing her that the divorce was not all her fault. Her stress and boredom diminished and her health improved with regular meals. As she began to regain control of her eating her bingeing and vomiting gradually stopped.

DO YOUR MOODS DICTATE YOUR EATING HABITS?

Breaking the link between your emotional state and your food intake can be the first step to successful weight control. Recognising that there is an emotional dimension to your eating may help you adopt healthier eating habits. By learning the triggers to your eating you can be prepared and either avoid these situations or have healthy snacks on hand. If you answer yes to one or more of these questions there may be an emotional factor affecting your eating habits.

QUESTIONS	YES	NO
Do you eat more when you are alone, for example, when watching television?		
Do you give yourself 'rewards' of chocolate or sweets if you've had a difficult day?		
If you've broken your diet and eaten a rich dessert, do you feel so upset that you might as well give up and eat what you like for the rest of the day?		
Does looking in the mirror or weighing yourself make you so depressed that you need a treat to cheer you up?		
Do you eat high-fat 'energy' foods, such as peanuts, crisps and chocolate, to give you a 'pick-me-up' boost when you're down?		

Yogic relaxation

Yogic techniques can reduce the stress that accompanies underlying problems related to food cravings and bingeing. Many community centres offer yoga classes and once you have learnt the basics, there will be many techniques, such as deep abdominal breathing (see below), that you can practise at home.

MUDRA BREATHING
Sit on your calves with back straight. Link your hands behind your back and push your shoulders back. Breathe deeply. On every second exhalation slowly lower the torso from the hips, for as long as the exhalation lasts; keep your back straight. As you inhale, slowly rise. Repeat four times.

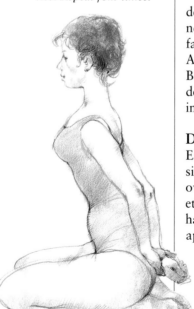

in 75 per cent of cases. A second study by Nicholas Troop at the Institute carried out from 1993 to 1995 found that women with eating disorders were less likely to respond well to stress and overcome the problems it posed than those without eating disorders.

It is often difficult to establish exactly what has caused the anxious or depressed state. The loss of a loved one, work pressure or relationship problems are obvious enough causes but anxiety and depression can also result from more deep-seated psychological problems that may need to be examined with the help of a professional counsellor.

Depression can in turn lead to nutritional deficiencies or imbalances as sufferers often neglect their dietary needs or turn to high-fat or sugary food for some sort of comfort. A lack of some micronutrients, particularly B vitamins and vitamin C, can contribute to depression and a vicious cycle of nutritional imbalance and depression may follow.

Dieting and depression

Early studies of women suffering from obesity suggested that the majority of sufferers overate directly in response to stress, anxiety and depression. Later studies, however, have indicated that the relationship between appetite, eating habits and emotional health is more complex than this. Research at the University of Toronto suggested that stress-induced overeating was actually a result of dieting. It was discovered that women who diet, and therefore restrain their desire for food, have two and a half times greater risk of developing eating disorders than non-dieters. Dieters tend to have strict rules about eating. For example there are many foods that are described as 'forbidden' – usually those that are high in fat or sugar. If they eat a forbidden food, they break a psychological rule which often leads them to decide that, as the diet is broken anyway, it may as well be forgotten until the next day when it can be started afresh. Breaking a diet rule can also contribute to a cycle of perceived failure, which in turn leads to a loss of self-esteem, and a comfort-eating response. Dieting itself can therefore contribute to the cycle of anxiety and overeating.

It can be very helpful to analyse your emotional state in relation to your food intake. Keeping a diary, for example, of what you ate and how you felt at the time may help you to pinpoint any emotional issues that need to be confronted. For example, did you eat a large number of biscuits while thinking about a relationship problem? Once you have established a link it is important to take steps to address the emotional problem. In the case of serious anxiety or depression consulting a counsellor may often be the best solution.

THE PSYCHOLOGY OF WEIGHT

For many people, body image becomes an obsession: impossible goals are set that can never be fulfilled. This leads to frustration, and depression at perceived failure. It is important to realise that your self-image is profoundly influenced by factors over which you have little control. Advertising images, models in magazines and on billboards, film and television stars, all embody ideals of beauty that most people find impossible to attain. However unrealistic we know these ideals to be, it's difficult to be immune to such influences at a subconscious level.

There has been a great deal of research on the topic of body image, and how women in particular often take an exaggeratedly negative view of their own bodies. Studies have shown that in general women think they are heavier than they really are, whereas men have a more accurate assessment of their body shapes. It is also interesting to note that women's perception of the most desirable female figure tends to be significantly thinner than the most desirable figure nominated by men, and more importantly, it is thinner than most doctors would recommend for optimal health.

Because some women so rigidly apply society's 'thin' messages to themselves, their self-esteem becomes almost entirely based on their body size and this increases their risk of developing eating disorders. In order to achieve realistic weight goals it is important to establish or to reclaim a sense of yourself as an individual, and not as a reflection of the role that society's current fashion dictates.

EATING DISORDERS

Two extreme and well-known examples of abnormal eating behaviour are anorexia nervosa and bulimia nervosa. Both these disorders involve an over-concern with weight and shape and an obsessive effort to lose weight over a long period of time, either by not eating or by indulging in inappropriate responses to food such as vomiting or using laxatives. The reasons why a distorted image develops are complex (see below), but some psychologists believe that much of the blame lies with the unrealistic images of beautiful women that bombard the public today, which particularly affect young women who are both more fashion-conscious and impressionable.

Anorexia nervosa is characterised by severe weight loss to the extent that a woman's periods will stop (they return once normal weight is regained). The other health risks include malnutrition, an increased risk of fracture due to osteoporosis, and, in extreme cases, death. Anorexics are often very secretive about their dietary habits, making treatment difficult.

continued on page 42

Dangerous ideals
The trend for extremely thin looking models went too far for a major watch manufacturer in 1995. The company threatened to suspend advertising from a top-selling British fashion magazine in response to its use of extremely thin models. One of the models, with a height of 1.75 m (5 ft, 9 in) weighed only 48 kg (7½ stone).

WHAT CAUSES EATING DISORDERS?

Eating disorders such as anorexia and bulimia nervosa are the result of complex and poorly understood causes. Sexual and mental abuse, parental conflict, pressure from sports coaches and the influence of society's ideals of body shape have all been implicated. As shown in the summary below, the sufferer falls into a cycle of depression and low self-esteem, which they express through an obsession with their weight. Once they start to link body image and eating with mood and self-esteem, a cycle of extreme dieting and/or bingeing and subsequent self-loathing can result. They may see weight loss as the solution to their problems and feel that exerting strict control over their diet will help them control their emotional difficulties. All eating disorders are potentially dangerous. Sufferers are unlikely to help themselves, and often deny having a problem. It is very important to break this negative cycle and professional help may be needed.

DISTORTED PERCEPTION
Social pressures and emotional problems can make a person of normal body weight perceive themselves as overweight.

| Stress, depression, low self-esteem. Morbid obsession with fatness. | Severe dieting. Overactivity. Obsession with exercise. | Severe weight loss. Fatigue, weakness. Poor skin and hair. Continued obsession with weight. | Uncontrolled binge eating followed by induced vomiting. | Severe psychological disorders – professional advice is needed. |

Clinical Psychologist

Clinical psychologists treat a range of disorders, including psychiatric depression, anxiety and eating problems and behavioural disorders, as well as some mental illnesses such as schizophrenia and manic depression.

REGULATING EATING PATTERNS
It is important for everyone to establish a balanced diet based on regular meals. People with eating disorders often skip meals in an attempt to eat less, and then end up bingeing later in the day because of hunger. Eating regular meals can be the first step on the road to recovery. Meals should be of moderate size and of healthy content so that they do not prompt any after-eating guilt responses.

Clinical psychologists may train in several areas of psychology, including psychotherapy. Their aim is to help people find their own solutions to problems such as relationship difficulties, binge eating or phobias. They are essentially concerned with a patient's current situation, but may ask about problems in the past if this seems relevant to the person's behaviour. Their questions are aimed at uncovering how patients think about themselves, their problems and goals. Treatment then tries to change the way that they think in order to help them change their behaviour. Because of the focus on thoughts (cognitions) and behaviour, one standard form of treatment is called cognitive-behavioural therapy.

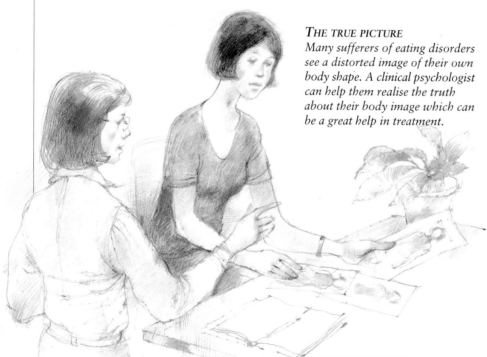

THE TRUE PICTURE
Many sufferers of eating disorders see a distorted image of their own body shape. A clinical psychologist can help them realise the truth about their body image which can be a great help in treatment.

What is the difference between a clinical psychologist and a psychiatrist?
A clinical psychologist is someone who has been trained in a number of psychological techniques which have a practical application for different psychological problems. All qualified clinical psychologists must meet requirements set out by the British Psychological Society but cannot prescribe drugs unless they have a medical degree.

A psychiatrist first obtains a medical degree and then specialises in psychiatric disorders, generally treating them with drugs. For eating disorders, however, psychological treatments are usually more effective than drugs. Because of this there is likely to be little difference between clinical psychologists and psychiatrists in practice, although a psychiatrist still has the option of prescribing drugs.

Do I need a referral from my GP?
This is the usual route, although other health professionals can refer you, for example a dietitian or counsellor. In the United Kingdom, however, funding for treatment is often held by GPs and so they need to approve the referral. If your GP is not a fundholder, he or she will still need to negotiate with the Health Authority to fund the treatment. If you feel unable to talk to your GP or he or she is reluctant to refer you (without giving you a satisfactory explanation), then change your GP to one who can help.

What will I need to talk to the psychologist about?

This question is difficult to answer in general terms as it depends on the specific treatment you have. The most usual form of treatment is cognitive-behavioural therapy which is concerned with symptoms, so the psychologist will generally want to know about your eating habits and your thoughts about weight and shape. You may be asked to complete a number of homework tasks to help in your treatment, such as keeping a food diary or writing a list of arguments for and against regaining control of eating habits to help motivation. Problems other than an eating disorder, like relationship difficulties, may also be relevant.

Some therapists may ask about problems that you might have had as a child and aim to resolve these in an attempt at overall treatment. It is up to you how much you tell the psychologist. You should remember, though, that the psychologist is there to help and, if you are not honest, he or she will have an incomplete picture of your problem and so may not be able to help as effectively.

How long will I need to see a therapist and how often?

A general course of treatment is usually between 16 and 20 sessions. More or less may be recommended depending on how severe your problem is. Initially, you may be asked to attend a couple of times a week. Later sessions may be spaced farther apart. The frequency of sessions will be negotiated between you and the psychologist. If you have not improved significantly within the initial course of treatment, you may be offered more sessions.

Will I need to see anyone else during treatment?

This depends on the nature of your problem and the resources available in the clinic. Options include a dietitian to help devise a sensible eating plan, family therapy if you are young and still live at home with your parents, or even group therapy with other sufferers.

Irrespective of the facilities available, your GP may be kept informed by your psychologist so that he or she may offer additional support or medical help.

Origins

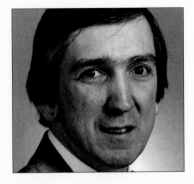

Professor Christopher Fairburn at Oxford University has led the development of the two most frequently used treatments for bulimia nervosa – cognitive-behavioural therapy (CBT) and interpersonal therapy (IPT). CBT is most widely used and aims to alter the negative thoughts that contribute to bulimia by regaining control over eating and modifying concerns about weight, shape and dieting. Many bulimia sufferers have problematic relationships with parents or partners and IPT largely focuses on these issues.

WHAT YOU CAN DO AT HOME

Here are two self-help methods you can try in conjunction with your professional treatment to help relieve your worries between sessions:

▶ *People with eating disorders often weigh themselves constantly. But as weight fluctuates naturally by a few pounds every day because of changes in fluid retention, this should not be taken to indicate long-term weight gain. Try to limit weighing yourself to once a day, at the same time each day. Work up to once a week. As your eating pattern normalises, you are likely to find that your weight also stabilises (though day-to-day fluctuations will continue).*

▶ *One way to increase both your motivation and optimism is to write two letters as if it were five years in the future. The letter could be to yourself, a friend (but do not send it) or someone* *imaginary. In the first letter, write as if you still have the eating problems – write about how you feel, what life with the eating disorder has been like over the last five years, for example, and the effects on your self-esteem, your health or your relationships. In the second letter, write as if you have recovered completely. Write about how you feel, acknowledge how difficult it may have been but also about the benefits that have occurred as a result of recovery, such as in your lifestyle and relationships. These letters should be as detailed and personal as possible.*

WRITING RELIEF
Writing a letter can allow you to release your true feelings. It will focus your mind on your problem, and boost your motivation by helping you envisage success.

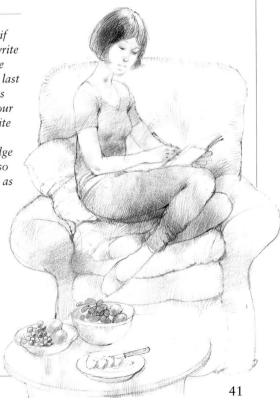

It may be less easy to identify those suffering from bulimia because they tend to be of normal weight. Bulimics have periodic uncontrollable binges usually followed by self-induced vomiting, abuse of laxatives or diuretics, fasting, obsessive exercising, and drug taking, for example, diet pills and amphetamines, in an attempt to get rid of the calories and avoid weight gain. The health risks of bulimia nervosa, although generally less severe than those of anorexia, are nevertheless serious. They include dehydration and loss of potassium, causing symptoms such as weakness and cramps. The gastric acid in vomit may also damage teeth and the lining of the throat.

Causes of anorexia and bulimia

Anorexia nervosa has been recognised for centuries but bulimia nervosa was first described in 1979 by Professor Gerald Russell, then at the Institute of Psychiatry in London. It is hotly debated whether the number of women with anorexia nervosa has increased over the years but it is almost universally accepted that the numbers of women with bulimia nervosa has increased since the 1960s with the rise of the diet culture and the number of women with bulimia is now far greater than the number with anorexia. Men also suffer from both diseases but to a far lesser extent.

Many people today blame the image of the supermodel and the craze for 'waif-like' female bodies for eating disorders, particularly among younger women. Whether or not these accusations are just – and the extent to which weight-reducing diets encourage eating disorders is unknown – these are certainly not the only causes. There are many other factors. These can include emotional difficulties during childhood such as sexual abuse, a difficult relationship with parents, neglect, and problems that arise during adulthood; low self-esteem, emotional and relationship problems and a fear of sex.

Few women develop bulimia nervosa in its most severe form. When extreme the disorder lies at the far end of the line of eating problems. However, some minor eating disorders may eventually lead to bulimia if the psychological problems behind them are not fully addressed, and many women show some of the same signs as bulimia sufferers, but at a much less severe level.

THE HEALTH RISKS LINKED TO ANOREXIA NERVOSA

Once body weight drops to a third or more below normal, signs of malnutrition, such as a gaunt, emaciated appearance, become evident. The normal hormonal balance is disturbed leading to thinning hair, bone wasting and an absence of periods. Poor vitamin and mineral intake causes deficiency disorders and disrupts the immune system, increasing risk of disease. Lack of body fat leads to rapid loss of body heat, sometimes to a life-threatening degree.

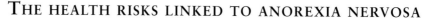

Hair gets thinner as a result of hormone changes and a lack of nutrients. At the same time, a fine downy hair (lanugo) may grow on the body

Breasts revert to pre-pubescent size because of muscle wasting, loss of body fat and hormone changes

Ovaries are affected by hormone imbalances leading to cessation of periods (amenorrhoea) and infertility

Skin gets very dry and nails become fragile because of disrupted hormone levels and poor diet

Bones become brittle and fracture easily (osteoporosis) as a result of reduced calcium intake and hormone imbalances

Teeth are gradually worn away by repeated self-induced vomiting, which causes decay, tooth loss and degeneration of the jawbone

Heart tissue is damaged by the low dietary intake of protein, vitamins and minerals, leading to irregular heartbeat and other cardiac disorders

Kidney damage and the risk of kidney failure result from long-term malnutrition

Muscles are broken down to provide vital energy in order to compensate for the low calorie intake, leading to muscle wasting

Intestines suffer long-term disruption to their digestive functions because of a lack of vital nutrients

LIFESTYLE FACTORS

Changes in the way we live our lives are emerging as the most significant reasons for the general increase in obesity in Western society over the past few decades.

Factors such as where, how and what we eat, combined with a decline in physical activity, have significantly affected the average weight of the population. In order to bring about a weight change it is necessary to resist the influences of society and in some cases, change your lifestyle towards healthier day-to-day living. The rate of increase in obesity in Western society is far too rapid to be accounted for by genetic factors. In the United Kingdom, for example, obesity in men rose from 6 per cent of the population in 1980 to 13.5 per cent in 1994; for women, the rise was from 8 per cent in 1980 to approaching 17 per cent in 1994.

LIFESTYLE AND WEIGHT

It is only over the last 50 years that people have had almost unlimited access to cheap calorie-dense food. Both takeaway food outlets and frozen or canned convenience foods from supermarkets have had a dramatic influence on the diet of the general population. These foods tend to be high in fats contributing to an overall calorie increase. The ease with which such foods can be bought and consumed has also encouraged the development of a 'snacking' culture where, rather than consuming regular balanced meals, people snack on nutritionally poor convenience foods. Children indulging in regular snacking is particularly worrying when as much as 45 per cent of their energy requirements may be eaten as snacks, often from high-fat foods such as crisps, chocolate and ice cream.

At the same time as dietary habits have changed, physical activity has also declined. Personal transport has increased and the technological revolution has outmoded many physically demanding jobs. Manual labour inside and outside the home has also been reduced. Leisure pursuits have become more sedentary with television watching becoming the most popular pastime for many people. The change in the health and fitness of the general population was highlighted in 1996 when the British army announced that its young recruits were failing fitness tests passed by earlier generations.

The effects of affluence

Like many chronic conditions, obesity appears to be more common among the poorer people of developed countries which suggests it relates to lifestyle factors. There is a strong correlation between social class and inactivity, and the relationship is stronger than that between social class and the amount of energy-foods eaten or the amount of fat consumed. While wealthier people tend to take more expensive steps towards improving their health and fitness such as enrolling at a gym, poor people tend to remain home-bound, particularly when they have young children, and television watching and similarly sedentary pursuits are often their primary leisure activities.

In developing countries the reverse is true. Individuals seem to be at higher risk of becoming obese the wealthier they become. This is probably due to a combination of factors, such as a reduction in exercise and

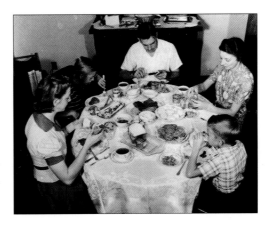

A FAMILY AFFAIR
One drawback to modern living is that families do not dine together as often as they used to. Try to make time for regular meals to reduce high-fat snacking.

the change to a higher-calorie diet, as they embrace the more sedentary lifestyle of an affluent society. The same is also true of migrant workers who move to more affluent countries; for example, Indian migrants to the United Kingdom.

Extensive entertaining and socialising also tends to be a feature of affluent societies. Eating out while on a weight-control plan can be a problem as many restaurants don't offer alternatives to their rich, exotic foods; add to this the temptations of desserts and alcohol and the goal of controlled, healthy eating becomes very difficult to achieve. But there are steps towards control which can be taken (see right).

Alcohol is not only high in calories, it also reduces your will-power. This means that after a few drinks it is easy to forget your good intentions and eat more than originally intended. Moreover, alcohol is an appetite stimulant so you are likely to eat more than usual if alcohol is served with your meal. Parties and pub or club nights can also be a problem because you are likely to be tempted to snack on calorie-laden, high-fat foods such as crisps.

Examining your lifestyle and quantifying how much exercise is undertaken in relation to the amount and type of food consumed, can be a sobering experience. It can also prompt you to find ways of introducing more activity into your daily life. Walking to the local shops, rather than taking the car, for example, could be the first step towards a more active lifestyle.

HEALTHIER SOCIAL EATING AND DRINKING

Going out for dinner needn't spell doom for your diet, and you don't have to avoid social events when trying to control your weight. These simple techniques can help you eat healthily.

▶ *Try to eat something nutritious and filling before going out to a party or for drinks, such as a meal of pasta and fresh salad. This will reduce the temptation to snack on unhealthy treats at the function and will give you energy to enjoy yourself.*

▶ *Choose restaurants which have low-fat, nutritious options on their menu. Remember, you can always ask the waiter for advice. Fish, grilled or steamed, is a good choice. You can also reduce the fat intake of a meal by removing skin from chicken before eating, or trimming fat from meat.*

▶ *Try to drink water some of the time while at the pub or at a party. This will not only control your alcohol intake, but will also help reduce the negative effects of alcohol such as dehydration.*

THE ROLE OF STRESS

Some stress can be beneficial when facing challenges; for example, a special project at work can be achieved with the help of some stress, because in small amounts it helps to concentrate and focus the mind. But too much stress can damage long-term health, reducing the efficiency of the immune system and leading to fatigue and illness.

Whether the physiological response to daily stress contributes to weight itself still remains unknown. In some cases stress may raise the metabolic rate as adrenaline raises the body's heart rate. Some people may also lose weight as their appetite decreases: digestive problems, often a symptom of stress, can lead to loss of appetite and weight. For some, the opposite can occur as comfort eating becomes a common response to stress, and weight gain results.

In either case, erratic eating behaviour, such as skipping meals or bingeing, tends to lead to eventual weight gain. Reducing daily stress can therefore be helpful in controlling weight. Regular exercise is a useful stress reliever or you could try relaxation techniques such as meditation or visualisation.

NUTRITIONAL VALUES OF SOME FAST FOODS

Many fast food meals are very high in fat (therefore delivering a lot of energy), yet offer little else of nutritional value. Although high-fat foods do fill you up, you tend to feel hunger pangs and a drive to eat much more quickly after eating them than if you had eaten foods that are high in carbohydrate.

FOOD	CALORIES	FAT (g)	CHOLESTEROL (mg)
Bacon and egg sandwich	427	22.7 g	246 mg
2 pieces extra crispy chicken	544	37 g	168 mg
Cola, 350 ml (12 fl oz)	136	0 g	0 mg
Quarter-pound burger	193	12.2 g	61 mg
Cheese and tomato pizza slice	235	11.8 g	16 mg
Milk shake, 350 ml (12 fl oz)	444	14 g	42 mg
French fries, regular size	280	15.5 g	0 mg

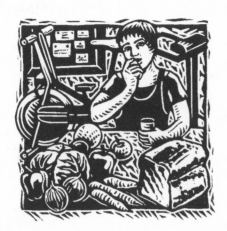

CHAPTER 3

MAINTAINING A HEALTHY WEIGHT

Controlling your weight can be a lot easier to manage if you understand why you feel the urge to eat. This chapter explains what your basic nutritional needs are, how to distinguish between hunger and appetite and how to handle the physiological and lifestyle changes that affect your weight from childhood through to old age.

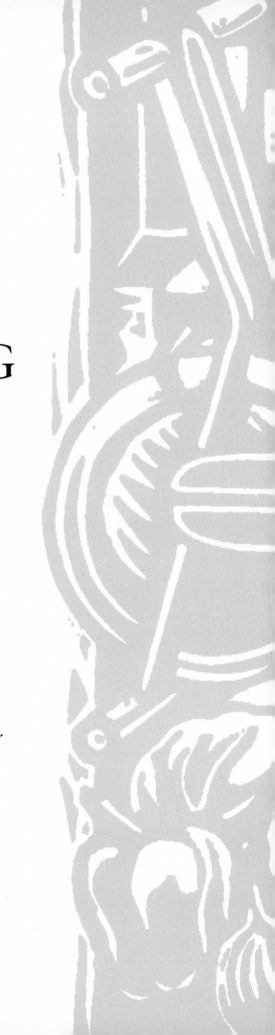

WHY WE EAT

Fuel is vital for our survival, for good health and for efficient functioning of the body. In modern Western society, however, we often turn to food for reasons other than true hunger.

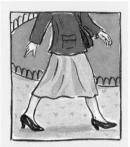

QUICK FITNESS TIP
If possible, walk part of the way to and from work. Alternatively, go for a brisk 20 minute walk at lunchtime.

The body has mechanisms to ensure an adequate intake of food (see page 28), but there are many other factors that can make you eat. Close-ups of food on television can stimulate your appetite; you might be bored or unhappy and use food as a comfort or a diversion; or you may be tempted to overeat at a dinner party.

FEELING HUNGRY

Hunger is the physiological need for food – the body's innate response to variations in its food supply. The body provides clear messages when it needs food: your stomach contracts producing a 'rumble'; in extreme cases you feel weak and faint. Appetite is the desire for food – a learned response to sensations or thoughts associated with food. It produces a number of physical effects, including increased salivation and the secretion of digestive juices in the stomach. An initial step in a weight-loss programme is to recognise the difference between these two states: to separate an urge for food from a need. Many things make you feel 'hungry' by sensually or psychologically stimulating your appetite. However, this does not mean that you are physically in need of food.

SOCIAL ENVIRONMENT

Food is one of the things that binds society together, and in most societies and cultures eating is among the most important social acts. All our major holidays and celebrations incorporate food as either the central celebration (for example the Christmas Day feast), or as an important part of the festivities such as the wedding or birthday cake. Relationships are cemented by food. Loved ones are taken out to dinner and lovers will even 'feed' one another as a sign of their affection. Friends meet over dinner and drinks, and in this context refusing food or alcohol can be interpreted as a snub. Business relationships are also strengthened by sharing food; weight is often a problem

---

FOOD FOR FEASTS AND FESTIVALS

Food has a spiritual importance in many faiths. Hindus, for example, worship the cow, and so hold butter and milk to be sacred. They also revere coconut because they believe its three 'eyes' symbolise their god Shiva. In Jewish tradition the house must be cleared of all leavened bread, which is made with yeast, before the Passover feast is celebrated. This festival marks the Israelites' escape from slavery in Egypt; while fleeing they were unable to prepare leavened bread as they could not wait for the dough to rise. Unleavened matzo bread is eaten during Passover, and is broken in two to symbolise Moses parting the Red Sea.

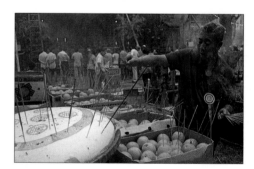

GIFTS FOR THE GHOSTS
During the Hungry Ghosts Festival, held in Hong Kong from mid-August to mid-September, offerings of food and other gifts are made to placate restless spirits who might otherwise take revenge on the living.

for a sales representative or self-employed business person who dines with clients to help build a trusting working relationship.

In any social environment we may feel pressure to eat more than we actually want or need in order to smooth interaction or foster a sense of camaraderie and goodwill. Once you have identified a link between overeating and social gatherings, however, you can start to make changes. Try not to schedule so many meetings – work or social – around mealtimes, and suggest other activities when you meet friends, such as going for a walk or playing some sport.

EMOTIONAL GRATIFICATION

We also eat for more complex emotional reasons (see page 36). We may eat because we are unhappy or depressed, because we're bored, or because we're stressed. Feeling 'full' can be warm and reassuring. A study of foreign students learning English in London in 1985 showed that feelings of homesickness lessened considerably while eating and immediately afterwards.

Other studies have shown that people who have been traumatised as children often turn to food for comfort and nurturing. These childhood habits can sometimes turn into a weight problem in adulthood. Comfort eating occurs in many different situations – at home, at work, in the car, at a social gathering; and for a variety of reasons – boredom, disappointment, dissatisfaction, loneliness, unhappiness, anger, or lack of confidence. Establishing how your emotions influence your eating patterns is crucial in maintaining healthy weight.

EATING FOR THE RIGHT REASONS

Diets will usually fail if food is used for comfort or as a diversion from other problems, but there are ways to minimise these impulses. To begin you need to write down in a diary or record book exact details of what you currently eat. Include 'hidden' foodstuffs such as mayonnaise on salads, and be scrupulously honest about between-meal snacks.

As well as writing down exactly what you ate, make a note of how you felt at the time. Were you unhappy or bored? And did this coincide with eating more biscuits than intended while watching television? Keeping this kind of diary will not only make you far more aware of exactly how much you really

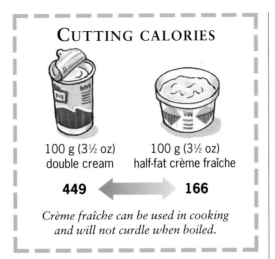

CUTTING CALORIES

100 g (3½ oz)
double cream

100 g (3½ oz)
half-fat crème fraîche

449 ⬌ **166**

Crème fraîche can be used in cooking and will not curdle when boiled.

consume during the day, it may also help you to establish if there is a pattern to your eating so that you can recognise any danger signs.

Your diary may reveal a few surprises. Research carried out in the UK in 1986 showed that obese women underestimated their food intake by an average of 800 calories a day. Another study in Holland in 1988 involving 525 men revealed that the most overweight individuals displayed the biggest discrepancy between actual calorie intake and estimated intake.

If your diary shows a link between boredom and snacking, in the first instance you will probably need to ensure you have low calorie snacks on hand such as fruit or rice cakes. In the longer term you should look at why you are feeling bored and what you can

---

BURNING OFF CALORIES: *Walking*

Walking is an ideal exercise for all ages. It is a good alternative to jogging, helping to develop cardiovascular fitness with far less risk of injury. For maximum aerobic benefit, maintain a brisk pace.

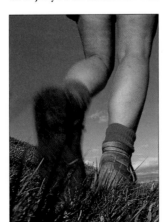

MUSCLE GROUPS BENEFITING
Regular walking will firm up all the leg muscles – especially those in the thigh and calf.

EQUIPMENT
Thick socks and a stout pair of walking shoes with good ankle support will help guard against blisters and sprains.

CALORIES BURNT
At 3 miles per hour, you burn 5 calories per minute: that's 300 calories per hour.

do to change these feelings. You could, for example, consider joining an evening class after work instead of watching television.

Eating while watching the television may also distract you from realising how much food you are consuming – and stop you giving your food due appreciation. Sitting down to a meal at the table and eating slowly so that you savour the food you have prepared will help you to feel satisfied and properly fed, and may prevent snacking later in the evening.

Think about any habits that you connect automatically, such as sofa/video/biscuits; cold/comfort/hot chocolate; work/coffee/doughnut, then learn to 'interrupt' them with healthier alternatives. Sofa/video/fruit; cold/comfort/herbal tea; work/coffee/cereal bar. This has the effect of questioning your choice of foods while making beneficial changes to your existing behaviour pattern.

Avoid shopping on an empty stomach, and before any item goes into the trolley, ask yourself whether you really need it.

Some people find it helps to make a list – and stick to it. Before mealtimes you should also think about each food item that you are planning to eat to decide whether it is really necessary and whether there is a healthier alternative, such as one that is lower in fat.

Instead of comfort eating, look for an alternative treat such as a long soak in the bath, a home manicure or pedicure, booking a free makeover advice session, or buying a bunch of flowers. Going for a long walk, especially in picturesque surroundings, can also be relaxing.

If your cravings for food become very strong, try to keep yourself busy. Clear out a cupboard, for example, or reorganise your book, music or video collection; put on a favourite piece of music, or look at photographs that evoke happy memories. Write a letter to a friend you have not seen or spoken to for a long time, or phone someone for a chat. You could also tidy your wardrobe and mix and match your clothes to create new outfits.

THE HUNGER GAUGE

Rediscovering eating as a response to feeling hungry, and being more objective about how hungry you actually are when you eat, can be a major step on the way to successful long-term weight control. The hunger gauge below aims to help you measure how hungry you are. It is best to eat when you are only moderately

hungry and to stop eating when you feel satisfied but could eat a little more. It is important that your food intake adequately sustains you during the day so that from one meal to the next you do not become ravenously hungry. If you eat at level 1, when you are desperately hungry, you are at risk of overeating.

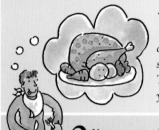

1 *You are desperately hungry and experiencing clear physical signs of hunger such as feeling faint and shaky. There is a risk of bingeing once you start to eat.*

2 *You are very hungry – your stomach is rumbling and you feel a little tired. You have waited just a little too long before eating and so there is still a risk of overeating.*

3 *You are moderately hungry; you have an appetite for food and a pleasant sense of anticipation – the ideal time to start eating. Only eat until you are satisfied and no more.*

4 *You feel satisfied. You could perhaps be tempted to eat dessert, but it's not essential. This is the ideal time to stop eating; aim to leave the table wanting just a little more and you will avoid feeling over full.*

5 *You are too full – you left it a little late to stop eating because you could not resist the temptation of another small helping and now you feel uncomfortable.*

6 *You are very full – you ignored all the signs to stop eating and now feel weighed down. You may also experience indigestion or heartburn.*

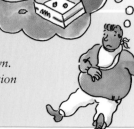

WHAT TO EAT TO STAY HEALTHY

The main purpose of eating is to provide the right fuel for your body to perform efficiently. Even when losing weight you should still be eating a healthy balance of foods.

Getting to know what your nutritional needs are, the role of different food groups and what constitutes a balanced diet makes good sense for your health: it can help you to adopt a nutritious diet and also to manage your weight.

FORMING A BALANCED DIET

The principle of healthy eating is balance: ensuring you eat the right amounts of carbohydrate, protein and fat from a variety of foods which provide essential vitamins and minerals. Complex carbohydrates (such as wholemeal bread, cereals, pasta, brown rice and potatoes) should make up the largest part of your diet. The next largest source of food should be vegetables and fruit, preferably raw or lightly cooked. Meat and dairy products are important for protein, but can be high in fat and so should be eaten in moderation. Finally, foods high in fats and sugars such as biscuits, cakes and chocolate, should be eaten sparingly.

CHANGING NEEDS

During your life there will be periods when your nutritional and calorie requirements have to adjust or change in response to different demands made upon the body.

Childhood

It is vital to understand the nutritional needs of a growing child. Infants and young children require energy for growth and so can eat more calorie-rich food than adults. Apart from children being generally more physically active, a child's metabolic rate is

continued on page 52

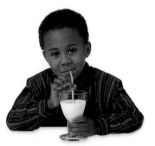

FOOD FOR GROWTH
Milk provides a rich source of calcium. Most nutritionists recommend that children should drink full-fat milk up to the age of five because they generally need the extra energy provided from the fat which is absent in low-fat milk.

UNDERSTANDING YOUR CALORIE NEEDS

To eat without putting on weight, you need to know your daily calorific needs. This can be calculated according to your gender, weight and level of activity. As shown below, the less active you are, the fewer calories you will need but as soon as you start to include a reasonable level of regular physical activity in your life your energy needs rise. Remember that your needs will be lower during periods of inactivity and you should reduce your calorie intake accordingly.

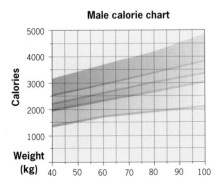

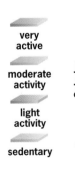

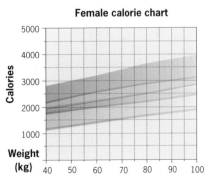

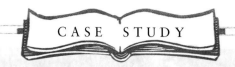

The Overworked Director

Leading a stressful, busy life in the 'fast lane' can lead you to adopt unhealthy lifestyle habits, such as eating high-fat foods, exercising infrequently or not at all, and smoking. In the long term, these habits can combine to produce potentially serious health problems. It is important to recognise what is happening and take the necessary steps to prevent further damage.

Andrew is a 44-year-old director and is married with two children. He has smoked an average of 20 cigarettes a day since his teens and now gets breathless going up stairs. He does no exercise other than taking his children to the park, and then only as often as his job permits. He is overweight, which he attributes to regular client entertaining. His work is pressured and he arrives home late every night, when he looks in on the children, has dinner (with wine) and then does his paperwork for the next day. In the morning he has a coffee and leaves for work very early. His father died at 55 from a heart attack as did his grandfather, but Andrew feels he has no time to do anything about his lifestyle.

WHAT SHOULD ANDREW DO?

Andrew needs to recognise that his lifestyle and genetic inheritance make him susceptible to heart disease, and he has to take steps to improve his lifestyle, starting with giving up smoking. He needs to delegate responsibility and prioritise his time to ease pressures at work, so that he can spend more time with his family and doing exercise. As dining with clients is part of his job, he needs to learn to select lower-fat alternatives from restaurant menus and cut back on his alcohol intake which will improve his performance at work, reduce calories and improve his health. Exercise relieves stress, and walking the children to school in the morning would also improve family relationships.

Action Plan

EATING HABITS
Cut back on the amount of fat and alcohol consumption within the diet to reduce the overall calorie intake.

FITNESS
Incorporate regular exercise into the daily routine to improve fitness, relieve stress and burn up excess calories.

WORK
Delegate work where possible, and prioritise the workload to allow adequate time for personal health and family commitments.

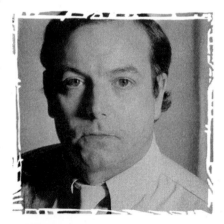

FITNESS
Busy people find it hard to make time for exercise during the day.

WORK
A demanding job places physical and emotional pressures on people.

EATING HABITS
A high-fat diet can cause high cholesterol and can damage the arteries. High alcohol consumption increases the risk of heart disease and hypertension.

HOW THINGS TURNED OUT FOR ANDREW

Andrew cut back his cigarettes and working lunches – only choosing low-fat options and soft drinks. He gave his staff more responsibility which alleviated some of his pressure, making him more effective at work. This meant he could leave later in the morning and walk his children to school. As family relationships improved, he spent more time with the children at the weekend, going for cycle rides regularly. In three months he had reduced his weight by 6.3 kg (1 stone).

WHAT MAKES A HEALTHY DIET?

There are seven essential nutrients that sustain human life: water, protein, carbohydrates, fats, vitamins, minerals and fibre. A healthy diet should include a balanced intake of all of these. Both excesses and deficiencies can be harmful to the body's health and efficiency. For example, not eating enough fruit and vegetables can lead to a weakening of the body's immune system. The food groups also interact; many people are not aware that excess protein can deplete calcium levels in the body. In order to help control your weight, look for foods that deliver little fat but provide other essential nutrients.

Water is the body's most basic nutritional need. It is required for almost every function: without it you will die in just a few days. It is important not to ignore thirst: some people try to lose weight by reducing fluid intake, but this is dangerous. As a general guide you should drink eight glasses of water daily. The body also gets water from food; milk, eggs, meat, vegetables and fruit all have a high water content.

Protein is produced from amino acids. It is essential for the growth and maintenance of body tissue, blood cells, hormones and enzymes. Protein is found in meat, poultry, fish, milk, cheese and eggs, vegetables such as green beans and tomatoes, grains, seeds and nuts. Ten to 15 per cent of your daily calorie intake should be from protein.

Carbohydrates provide fuel to meet energy needs. The most important carbohydrates are 'complex' carbohydrates, also known as starches. They are found in many plant foods such as wheat, rice, potatoes, pasta and yams. Carbohydrates should form 55 to 60 per cent of your diet.

Fibre is indigestible carbohydrate and is very important for general health; there are two types, insoluble and soluble. Insoluble fibre helps the digestive process; it can help prevent haemorrhoids and may also help protect against cancer of the lower bowel. Sources include wheat, rice, pasta, bran, wholegrain cereals and breads, nuts and prunes. Soluble fibre is thought to help reduce cholesterol, and thus help prevent heart and arterial disease. It is found in oats, peas, beans, root vegetables and citrus fruits. The recommended intake of fibre is 18 g per day.

Fat is essential as an energy store, to help insulate the body against rapid heat loss, help the body produce hormones, cushion vital organs such as the liver and kidneys, and aid the absorption of certain vitamins. Fat should represent about 30 per cent of the diet but most people eat much more. There are two main types of fats: saturated (such as butter) and unsaturated (such as vegetable oil). Foods very high in fat such as fast foods, fried foods and sugary snacks should be avoided as they offer little nutrient value. Unsaturated fats, on the other hand, may help protect against heart disease.

Vitamins are organic compounds, essential for bodily growth, function, repair and maintenance. Vitamins are categorised into two groups, water soluble and fat soluble. Water soluble vitamins, including the B complex group and vitamin C, need to be replenished daily as they are not stored in the body's tissues. Fat soluble vitamins, including A, D, E and K, are stored by the body for long periods of time, and so excessive intake may be harmful. A balanced diet with plenty of fresh fruit, vegetables and cereals should provide all the vitamins that the body needs.

Minerals are essential inorganic compounds that aid energy production and body maintenance as well as assisting in the control of body reactions and reflexes. There are three groups; macrominerals, microminerals and trace elements. Macrominerals including calcium, sodium and magnesium are required in large amounts. The body needs microminerals, which include iron, manganese and zinc, in lesser quantities. Trace elements required in minuscule amounts include manganese and iodine. A diet that provides a balance of lean red meat, fish, dairy products, nuts, cereals and pulses and a wide range of vegetables should provide all the minerals essential for health.

A BALANCED DIET – AS EASY AS 12345

The 1+2+3+4+5 plan provides a balanced daily diet. Each day, eat 1 piece of meat, poultry, seafood or meat substitute, 2 portions of dairy products, 3 pieces of fruit, 4 portions of vegetables, 5 servings of breads/cereals, plus a small treat. This menu shows how you can spread these portions throughout your day.

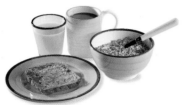

Breakfast
Muesli with semi-skimmed milk, orange juice, 1 slice wholemeal toast with low-fat vegetable spread, coffee with semi-skimmed milk = 1 portion dairy, 2 breads/cereals and 1 fruit

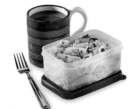

Lunch
Pasta with Italian green beans and sweetcorn and yoghurt dressing, coffee with semi-skimmed milk = 1 portion bread/cereal, 2 vegetable

Morning snack
Tea with semi-skimmed milk, 1 banana = 1 portion fruit, 1 dairy (the milk in all drinks and the spread on toast combine to make 1 dairy portion)

Dinner
Grilled steak, brown rice, steamed courgettes and carrots, garlic bread, and a trifle for dessert = 1 portion meat, 2 breads/cereals, 2 vegetables and 1 treat

Afternoon snack
1 apple = 1 portion fruit

also proportionally higher than an adult's, so energy is burnt off much faster. Young children should eat larger amounts of dairy products than adults as these are an ideal source of calcium and high-quality protein, both essential for healthy growth.

Children should never be put on a weight-loss plan as this can interfere with healthy growth. If your child is severely overweight, consult your doctor. You can help to establish healthy eating habits in your child; don't try to make a child finish a meal if they say they are full and don't give too large a portion. Children learn a lot from watching their parents so try to encourage healthy eating habits from a young age.

Teenagers

Because the body undergoes a growth spurt at puberty, many teenagers – boys, in particular – will feel constantly hungry. A boy's basal metabolic rate (BMR) will remain high until around age 20, so he will be able to eat more than he needs without putting on weight. A girl's BMR drops away much more quickly; by around age 15 it is generally at adult level. Neither adolescent boys nor girls should be encouraged to diet as they still have relatively high nutritional needs. But there is a danger today that teenagers may exceed their energy needs and end up overweight because of the wide range of high-fat fast foods available to them. It is therefore important to encourage them to adopt healthy eating practices.

During and after pregnancy

Pregnancy and breastfeeding both place special dietary demands on the body. Foods that are rich in iron and calcium should be increased in the diet; iron can help prevent birth defects; and calcium will be needed for the baby's bone development.

Many women date the start of weight problems to pregnancy but research shows that it is not because their metabolism has become sluggish after giving birth. Changes in lifestyle that follow childbirth such as eating more (especially snacks) and being less active are a likely cause of weight gain or the reason why weight gained during pregnancy is not lost. This can be overcome by exercise and by making dietary changes.

After pregnancy, most women weigh more than before they conceived. Breast-feeding may help to lose this excess weight

DID YOU KNOW?

Protein is vital for growing children. Between the ages of one and three, they need more than twice the amount of protein in relation to their size as an adult does. The amount needed decreases as the child gets older but children between seven and ten still need a third more total intake of protein in relation to their size than an adult.

if it is continued for at least six months; it also supplies the best source of nutrition for the baby.

Old age

While the elderly should continue to follow recommended adult guidelines for nutrition, particular health problems associated with ageing may be prevented or relieved by diet changes. Maintaining the intake of calcium will protect against osteoporosis, although if there is a family history of the disease, the best course is a high intake of calcium in adolescence and young adulthood. Iron (from red meat, cereals, vegetables and dried fruit) will be beneficial for red blood cell formation as anaemia can be a problem in old age, and increasing the amount of fibre will reduce constipation and maintain digestive tracts.

Unless an elderly person remains particularly active, they will not need as much energy as someone in their 30s, and reducing overall intake of fat is a wise precaution against heart disease and other problems associated with fat in the diet.

ALCOHOL AND WEIGHT

Specific lifestyle or physiological factors can also affect your nutritional needs. Smoking (see box below) and excessive drinking may deplete your body of essential nutrients.

Heavy drinkers sometimes suffer from nutritional deficiencies as their dependence on alcohol causes them to neglect their diet. The British government recommendations

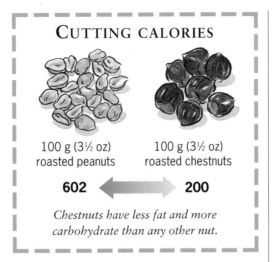

CUTTING CALORIES

100 g (3½ oz) roasted peanuts

100 g (3½ oz) roasted chestnuts

602 ⬅➡ **200**

Chestnuts have less fat and more carbohydrate than any other nut.

for maximum weekly levels of alcohol are 28 units for men and 21 for women. This is based on one unit being equivalent to one measure of spirits, a glass of wine, or half a pint of beer. If you drink in excess of these levels you may be damaging your health.

Alcohol has a high calorie content, but because it is toxic and cannot be stored by the body, it is converted to energy and used before dietary energy sources which can be stored. This means that drinking will encourage food to be stored as fat and hence weight is gained. Finally, alcohol weakens your will-power so that if you drink alcohol while on a diet you may forget your good intentions. Research shows that people eat more at meals consumed with alcohol than when alcohol is absent from the table. Any weight-management plan should aim to control alcohol intake.

TIPS FOR REDUCING ALCOHOL INTAKE

Any weight-loss plan will benefit greatly if you reduce your alcohol intake. Here are some suggestions on how you can achieve this:

▶ *Halve the money you take with you to the pub so that you cannot succumb to temptation.*

▶ *Drink ½ pint glasses of beer or lager instead of pints and try to make them last the same time.*

▶ *Drink single measures of spirits, not doubles.*

▶ *At a meal where wine is in abundance, have a jug of water on the table. When you are drinking for thirst, drink water instead of gulping wine.*

QUIT SMOKING AND AVOID WEIGHT GAIN

Everybody knows that smoking is bad for health but some people fear that if they quit they will gain weight. Smoking raises your metabolism, and when you stop, the energy you take in from food is burnt less efficiently. Furthermore, instead of eating less, many people eat high-fat snacks to replace cigarettes and weight gain results. This can be avoided with diet and lifestyle changes.

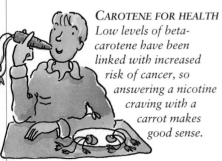

CAROTENE FOR HEALTH *Low levels of beta-carotene have been linked with increased risk of cancer, so answering a nicotine craving with a carrot makes good sense.*

▶ *Eat less fatty foods and replace them with 'tummy fillers' like rice and pasta.*

▶ *To boost your well-being and to make up for the drop in your metabolism when you give up smoking, begin an exercise regime. This can be as simple as going for a brisk 30 minute walk each day.*

▶ *Begin an evening course or start a new hobby to help re-focus your mind away from smoking and keep you busy at times when you might otherwise smoke.*

SUITABLE SNACKS *Vary your low-fat snacks. Try sticks of raw vegetable, fresh fruit, or a filling drink of fruit blended with low-fat yoghurt.*

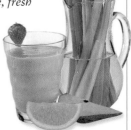

LIFELONG HEALTHY WEIGHT

Long-term successful management of weight means forming good habits from childhood onwards. Many studies show that childhood obesity can lead to a lifetime of weight problems.

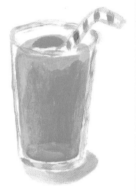

HOMEMADE FIZZ
Children love fizzy drinks but canned drinks usually contain high amounts of sugar as well as other additives such as caffeine. A healthier option is to make your own fizzy drinks at home using pure unsweetened fruit juice and carbonated water.

FAMILY OUTINGS
Days out that focus on fun but are centred around exercise will improve the fitness of all the family. Cycling trips in the countryside, long walks or a day at a local swimming pool with wave machines and slides will all provide good aerobic exercise that is fun for the whole family.

There is strong evidence to show that an overweight child often grows up to be an overweight adult. One reason for this might be that eating the wrong types of food and taking insufficient exercise at a young age are difficult habits to break as you grow up.

CHILDREN'S WEIGHT

Alarmingly, the number of overweight and obese children is growing rapidly – some studies suggest the number of significantly overweight children in Britain doubled in the 20 years between 1960 and 1980. The role of parents in promoting a healthy lifestyle is crucial. Statistics show that if a child has an obese parent the child will have a 40 per cent chance of becoming obese also. The risk is doubled if both parents are obese.

If parents are uninformed or casual about healthy eating and undertake little exercise they are introducing their children to the lifestyle risks for obesity. Setting a good example, by eating well and taking regular exercise, is essential to teach children a

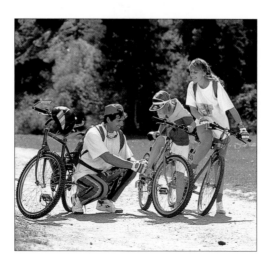

proper respect for their body. Using food as a method of behavioural control can also develop the wrong attitudes about diet in children. If sweets are given as a reward for good behaviour and children are told they must eat up their vegetables in order to get dessert, messages are being sent about 'nice' and 'nasty' food at a very early age.

Being creative in meal planning can be a way to introduce healthier foods subtly into the family's diet. Most children enjoy the natural sweetness of fresh fruit, and a fresh fruit salad served with low-fat yoghurt is an appealing dessert. Disguising healthy food as 'fast food' can also be very successful: homemade hamburgers using wholemeal buns, grilled burgers made with high quality lean mince, fresh tomato and lettuce provides a healthy meal. It can also be helpful to try gradually reducing the amount of salt and sugar added to recipes – children will probably resist dramatic changes but may fail to notice a slow but steady decline.

Exercise needs to be introduced as an integral part of the family's lifestyle. Watching television and playing video or computer games should be balanced with more active pursuits. Many parents are anxious about their children playing unsupervised in parks and in the street, but some sociologists believe that increased levels of fear in our society have led to a cocooning mentality where the home is considered to be the only safe place for children. Encouraging children to join youth clubs and supervised sporting organisations can be a way to reduce this concern.

If children don't like sport (this can often be a problem with overweight or self-conscious children), joining a non-sporting club
continued on page 58

Middle-Age Spread

As people age their metabolism slows down and their body burns less energy. In addition, older people often live a sedentary lifestyle. But middle-age spread needn't be inevitable. Changing your diet to avoid fat and increasing your level of activity will both help to control weight. These changes will have positive benefits for your health too, guarding against many diseases.

As you age your calorie requirements decrease slightly because your resting metabolic rate is lower. Since fewer calories are burned, more will be stored as fat. Another effect of ageing is that people become less active. The body tends to lose muscle and since muscle burns more energy than fat, this further reduces the body's energy needs. There are two ways of counterbalancing these effects. The first is to increase your exercise level so that your body stems the loss of muscle and burns more fat, and the second is to look at your diet and find ways of eating more healthily and decreasing the amount of energy in the diet.

TIPS TO IMPROVE YOUR DIET

You can consume fewer calories without eating a smaller volume of food if you choose lower fat items. You should also plan your eating to boost your metabolism. Don't skip meals as this will cause your metabolism to be sluggish all day and then, if you eat a large meal later to compensate, it cannot burn off all the extra calories consumed. Breakfast is especially important because it acts as a kick start to your metabolism which slows during sleep.

▶ *Change to low-fat dairy alternatives.*
▶ *Use low-fat spreads instead of butter and cut back the amount you use.*
▶ *Choose lean cuts of meat. Trim off any visible fat. Remove the skin from poultry after cooking.*

COOKING BY STEAM
Steaming vegetables ensures that more vitamins are retained. Spread the raw vegetables out in the steamer so they cook evenly.

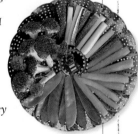

WARMING UP

Exercise will have benefits for your general health, helping to maintain joint flexibility and mobility, and can help ease some of the symptoms of arthritis. Look at the type of exercise you are doing – if it is painful, there may be a better alternative. Swimming can be very beneficial as it supports your weight allowing freer movement of joints and muscles. Warming up is vital before more vigorous exercise, or it can be used as a daily routine to ease you from sedentary habits into an exercise plan.

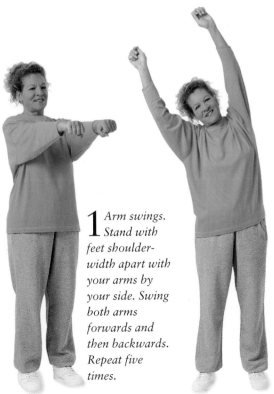

1 *Arm swings. Stand with feet shoulder-width apart with your arms by your side. Swing both arms forwards and then backwards. Repeat five times.*

2 *Body stretches. Stand with your feet shoulder-width apart. Raise both hands over your head and lean gently to your right while still facing the front. Repeat, leaning gently to the left. Stretch five times for each side.*

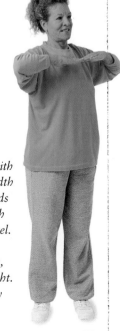

3 *Back swings. Stand with your feet shoulder-width apart and clasp your hands in front of your chest with elbows bent and arms level. Slowly rotate your upper body to the left five times, and then repeat to the right. Keep your hips stationary during the exercise.*

The PE Teacher

A good physical education teacher will motivate children to take an interest in sport and fitness, giving them the right start for a healthy adult lifestyle. Understanding educational approaches may help you to encourage your own children to be more active.

THE INSTRUCTOR
Over the last decade the incidence of child obesity has rocketed, and the decline of team sports and physical education has to some extent been blamed. Today's PE teacher has a difficult task. He or she has to motivate children to take an interest in sport when, due to today's more sedentary lifestyle, they may be lacking in fitness and enthusiasm.

SHOWING THE WAY
A PE teacher is responsible for ensuring that children know how to exercise safely without damaging growing muscles. A guided warm up at the start of the class and cool down at the end are essential.

Educationalists today recognise the importance of establishing healthy lifestyles for children, but they are also aware of the vital role of motivation. Much of the current thinking behind physical education programmes focuses on getting every child directly involved. Small group games are encouraged rather than large whole class games so that no child misses out on participating. Even if a child is unable to take an active part in the lesson, he or she is still encouraged to attend and help to plan activities or evaluate other children's work.

What qualifications do you need to become a physical education teacher?
Entrance into PE teaching is possible through a number of routes, but as teaching is now nearly an all-graduate profession, you generally need a degree. It could be a Bachelor of Education or it could be within another discipline followed by a postgraduate certificate of education. A Bachelor of Education with Physical Education as the main subject is usually a four-year honours course. Students learn about physiology and health, human movement, education and teaching practices. It is also possible to take the degree with PE options at both primary and secondary level.

What sort of clothing should children wear?
Most schools will have a PE uniform of shorts and short-sleeve tops; sometimes gym skirts for the girls. Plimsolls or trainers are important footwear, and track suits are encouraged for outdoor games and athletics, particularly in cold winter months. Children should not wear jewellery during sport as this can increase the chance of injury.

What activities are children taught at school?
Children are taught at various degrees of complexity and intensity throughout their primary and secondary years, starting off at the simplest levels of participation and understanding and gradually building

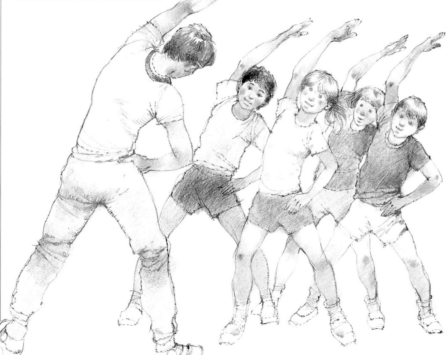

up to more advanced levels of individual and team competition. In the United Kingdom the physical education curriculum is structured around six main activities aimed at providing a broad range of exercise experience: games, gymnastic activities, dance, athletic activities, swimming, and outdoor and adventure activities. All of these aim to build children's fitness levels and motor (or movement) skills, but some areas have specific additional areas of focus. Games for example, aims to develop co-operation and communication with others, as well as concepts of fair play and the application of rules. Gymnastics, on the other hand, is specifically aimed at developing controlled body movement, strength and flexibility. Dance tries to help children learn about movement as a medium for expression, while athletics focuses on particular motor skills such as running, jumping and throwing. Swimming develops breathing techniques and particular muscle groups. Finally, outdoor and adventure activities give children a chance to face and overcome challenges in a natural environment, building confidence and initiative. Adventure activities are also particularly good for increasing enthusiasm and motivation.

All six of these areas of activity are designed to increase children's awareness of the general themes of health and fitness, meeting personal and group challenges, and developing a positive attitude to physical activity.

How does a teacher develop interesting activities for children of different age groups?

Teachers aim to structure activities to match the psychological and physical stage of development of the child. For example, in a games class for seven-year-olds the children would be taught to develop their skills in throwing and catching, and playing easy games like 'Piggy in the Middle'. Complicated rules and skills might be too difficult for younger children to understand and could result in the loss of their interest. At age 10 children are introduced to particular skills such as controlling a ball while moving, and to new concepts such as marking an opponent. Not until they are 11 or 12 years old are children expected to take part in formal games such as football, netball or hockey, and teams are still kept to small numbers (perhaps four a side) so that all the children learn the basic principles. In dance classes, nine-year-olds are taught ideas about contrasting movements, for example travelling, turning or making arm gestures; at age 10 they start to learn about moving in set patterns, following one movement with another; and by the age of 12 they are learning how to move and shape the body to suggest a certain character or an emotion.

How do teachers motivate reluctant children?

Teachers use a lot of patience to encourage reluctant or embarrassed children to take part in activities, but they must not ignore the needs of the rest of the class. Situations where a child feels self-conscious or inadequate should be avoided. Instead they can be put into 'easy' situations within teams of children with mixed sporting ability so that they do not feel useless or unwanted. They can help develop rules for a game, for example, or adapt existing rules to make a game fairer. By giving children tasks at which they can succeed, their confidence is boosted and a positive attitude is fostered. Teachers try to develop an atmosphere of support during lessons so that children of every level can enjoy themselves without fear of negative criticism or undue pressure.

WHAT YOU CAN DO AT HOME

Try to build on your child's enthusiasm for a particular school sport. Encourage your child to attend after-school sports practice sessions if they get picked for a team, and always try to be there to support them when parents are invited to watch. You could also investigate community clubs in your area that your child could join after school. Many clubs offer coaching and skills development to improve a child's proficiency. It might also be helpful to look at ways in which the whole family can share an activity so that everyone exercises together – which is good for your activity level as well as theirs. If your child enjoys dancing, for example, there might be local dance nights that the family could attend together. Getting the whole family involved will reinforce what your child is learning at school, and show your support and pride in what they are achieving. This can help to increase their confidence, which in turn will improve their ability and enjoyment.

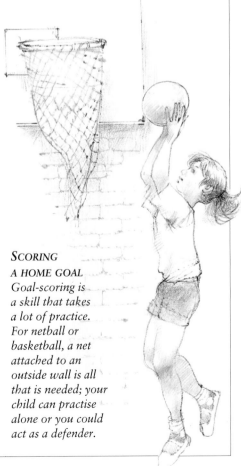

SCORING

A HOME GOAL
Goal-scoring is a skill that takes a lot of practice. For netball or basketball, a net attached to an outside wall is all that is needed; your child can practise alone or you could act as a defender.

DIET AND THE ELDERLY

Elderly people have conflicting dietary needs. On the one hand they need fewer calories and less volume of food than they did in their younger days, but on the other hand they require just as many nutrients. The food they eat, therefore, must be nutrient dense to provide all the necessary elements – especially calcium, vitamins and fibre.

But older people may have neither the budget nor inclination to cook elaborate dishes with costly ingredients. A salad of monkfish, kale and pine kernels may be fine for entertaining, but is hardly practical for day-to-day cooking.

Soups provide the necessary combination of convenience, nutrient density and low price. A blender or a food mill is all that is required to turn everyday ingredients into a filling, healthy dish. Home-made soups have a distinct advantage over canned ones. Using fresh, unprocessed ingredients will allow you to control levels of salt and sugar, and preserve nutrients that are lost in processing. Try pea soup, made with frozen peas, onion, some lettuce, mint and yoghurt and some water. You could also substitute vegetables like broccoli or carrots for the peas.

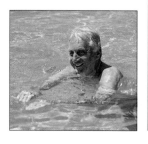

EXERCISE AND AGE
Regular exercise is very important for the elderly – it can prevent the weight gain that often accompanies a slower pace of life after retirement, and helps to keep bones strong and joints supple.

can still be beneficial. Drama or art may not promote fitness to the same extent as sporting activities, but research shows that almost any activity burns more calories than television watching. Children will also be far less tempted to eat while taking part in an outside activity than while sitting watching the television, which encourages snacking, often of high-fat, unhealthy foods.

When trying to change children's diet and exercise habits it is important to avoid criticism and to offer support and encouragement at all times. Children need to feel that good dietary habits and exercise are enjoyable and positive rather than associated with negative feelings. It is also possible to make a child obsessive about weight to the point where children as young as six and seven place themselves on diets. Balance and proportion is the key, and gradual rather than dramatic changes provide the best long-term results.

AVOIDING WEIGHT GAIN THROUGH LIFE

Many people gain weight as they age. But recent research has shown this needn't be inevitable. While the body's metabolic rate does slow down after the mid to late 30s, the main reason why people gain weight seems to be due to a reduction in exercise and general levels of activity.

For women, the menopause also leads to changes in fat distribution due to a drop in the level of oestrogen (see page 19). At this time of life, fat begins to collect around the waist and on the stomach.

By understanding that the body now needs fewer calories you can make changes at this crucial time and prevent or at least reduce weight gain. Stopping weight gain before it happens will involve far less effort than trying to lose weight later on.

Try to stay as active as possible as you get older – exercise is still a major factor in a healthy life, helping to increase joint mobility and alleviate the symptoms of arthritis. In fact, you should be more active during middle age to burn off the extra calories that your slower metabolism is not using.

You should also make dietary changes – cut down on high calorie foods, those high in fat and sugar with little nutritional value, and increase your level of complex carbohydrates. As you grow older, you may find it hard to digest three main meals and prefer to take a 'little and often' approach.

Knowing your needs

Identifying your specific nutritional needs and adapting your food intake accordingly is a lifelong commitment. If for example, you become ill and are bedridden, the nutritional value of your food needs to be high but your calorie intake requirements will be reduced as you are completely inactive. If you are short of time and find it difficult to include exercise or activity in your day, a similar adjustment should be made. Conversely, it is important to maintain a healthy weight and not let your weight fall too low as you age – evidence suggests that fractures associated with osteoporosis are more likely among thin women.

CHAPTER 4

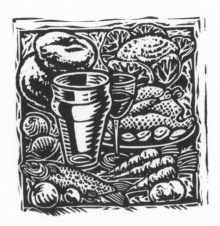

FOODS AND YOUR WEIGHT

*It is hardly surprising that so many people find it
hard to lose weight when the popular image of a
diet is obsessive calorie counting and tiny portions
of an unappetising food. But by changing the
balance of the different types of food you eat you
can lose weight – or gain it if you need to – and
still enjoy your meals, without the need to
weigh every mouthful.*

FOOD TYPES AND YOUR WEIGHT

For successful weight control, it helps to be aware of the varying effects that different food groups, such as proteins, carbohydrates and fats, have on your appetite and your weight.

When trying to lose weight, you need to choose foods that are low in calories while delivering a high level of nutrients. But if your weight-control plan is to be successful, it doesn't stop there. To keep your motivation going, you will need to make sure your meals are tasty and enjoyable and that they fill you up and don't leave you feeling hungry. Otherwise the temptation to reach for a high-fat, high-sugar snack will be too strong.

WHAT FOODS FILL YOU UP?

Many people can successfully introduce healthy, low-fat main meals into their diet, but find that they still crave dessert, even if their stomach is full. This is because the part of your brain that controls appetite may register satisfaction from one type of food but still signals appetite if a different type of food is on offer. This is why a glimpse of the sweet trolley, or the waitress asking if anyone would like dessert is often enough to persuade you that you are still hungry.

Another reason why you may still feel like dessert after eating a perfectly satisfying main course is that it takes time for food to digest and be converted to energy in the body. If you wait about half an hour after a main course you will feel less like eating anything else. Similarly, you will also be less likely to want second helpings if you wait for a while after the first serving.

Fats versus carbohydrates

Many studies have shown that foods that are low in calories for their weight and high in fibre and water, such as baked potatoes, fill you up more quickly than those high in calories for their weight and low in fibre and water, such as croissants. Similarly, while many people love to eat fatty foods like chips, high-fat foods are less effective at filling you up than high carbohydrate foods and eating them can lead to 'passive over-consumption' (see page 29). If you eat fatty foods you need to eat more calories to achieve the same sense of fullness and satisfaction than if you eat high carbohydrate foods. So, if you are trying to control your weight or to lose weight, you should increase complex carbohydrates in your diet,

DIETARY PROPORTIONS

Eating a balanced diet means eating the right proportions of each food type. The illustrated section of this chart shows the percentage of carbohydrates, protein and fats that should make up your daily diet. The outer plain-coloured section shows, on average, what most people actually do eat.

Carbohydrates should form 55 to 60 per cent of your daily diet

Fats should make up no more than 30 to 35 per cent of your daily diet

Protein should make up about 10 to 15 per cent of your daily diet

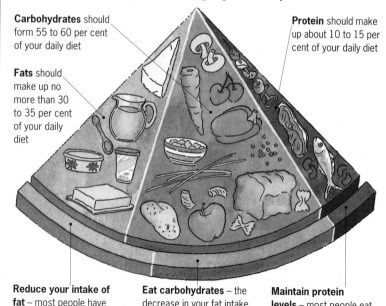

Reduce your intake of fat – most people have about 10 per cent too much fat in their diet

Eat carbohydrates – the decrease in your fat intake can be replaced by eating more carbohydrates

Maintain protein levels – most people eat about the right amount of protein

CUTTING CALORIES

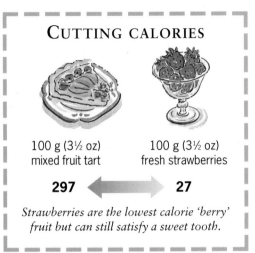

100 g (3½ oz) mixed fruit tart

100 g (3½ oz) fresh strawberries

297 ◄──────► **27**

Strawberries are the lowest calorie 'berry' fruit but can still satisfy a sweet tooth.

such as potatoes and wholegrains, as well as fruits and vegetables which are filling but contain relatively few calories, and cut down on sugary, high-fat foods which are high in calories but don't fill you up.

In this way you can significantly reduce your daily calorie intake. A good example is breakfast. If you have a high-fat breakfast, such as two croissants with butter and jam, you are much more likely to want a mid-morning snack than if you eat a more healthy breakfast, say a bowl of bran flakes and some toast. In the same way at lunchtime have an apple as your final snack instead of, for example, a bag of crisps. Apples are high in fibre and water and should fill you up much more effectively.

PROTEINS AND YOUR WEIGHT

Protein is the major structural material of the body. It is vital for the maintenance of cells, tissues and organs, for muscle strength, and the health of your hair, skin and nails. It is also the major component of the enzymes and hormones that regulate the body's metabolism.

When protein is digested, it is broken down into its constituent building blocks known as amino acids. These are transported around the body to be used as needed. The remainder of the protein molecule is essentially sugar and this is used either for energy – it provides 4 calories per gram, the same as carbohydrates – or stored as glycogen in the liver and muscles.

Daily requirements of protein differ with individual needs. For example, protein needs are higher for children, athletes, and people suffering from illness or disease. Protein intake should also be increased during pregnancy and breast feeding. Your daily intake of protein should be 10 to 15 per cent of your total calorie intake.

High protein foods include lean meats, poultry, beans and pulses, eggs and dairy foods. Be careful, however, because protein rich foods are often high in fat, and too much protein accelerates calcium excretion. If you are eating sufficient protein there is no evidence that eating more will build up muscle without added exercise. Instead, the

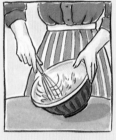

QUICK FITNESS TIP
Instead of using labour-saving devices like food processors and electric mixers, burn some calories by chopping, blending and whisking by hand.

NEGATIVE CALORIE FOODS

No food contains negative calories – that is, burns more calories in being digested than it actually provides itself. However, some foods, such as celery, contain very few calories, so you can eat as much as you like without putting your weight-control programme at risk.

Most fruits and vegetables are very low in calories (see page 67) so they are an important part of any weight-control programme. Packed with vitamins and minerals, they make healthy snacks which can help you to stave off hunger pangs. By filling up on vegetables you are more likely to be able to resist the temptation to eat sugary, high-fat snacks which are loaded with calories and yet offer little or no nutritional value.

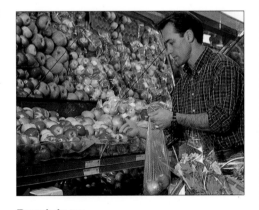

PICK 'N' MIX
Try a variety of fruits and vegetables. Many supermarkets now stock exotic types like yam or cassava as well as familiar favourites. Keep a supply of frozen vegetables in the freezer so you don't run short.

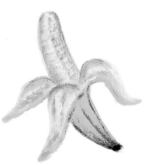

CHOOSE A BANANA
Bananas are a healthy choice if you crave something sweet. Although they are higher in calories than other fruits, they are also high in complex carbohydrates and fibre and are therefore more filling. They also provide important vitamins and minerals including potassium, zinc, iron, folic acid and calcium.

extra protein will be used to provide energy – and the fat you eat, rather than being used for energy, will be stored.

CARBOHYDRATES AND YOUR WEIGHT

Carbohydrates are essential for health, their main function being to provide energy for the body – one gram provides four calories. Many important vitamins and minerals are also found in high-carbohydrate foods.

Complex carbohydrates, such as potatoes, rice, pasta, wholegrain cereals and breads, should form the largest part of a healthy diet, particularly one that aims to control weight. They contain fibre which fills you up (helping to prevent overeating), help to maintain an efficient digestive system, lower cholesterol levels and protect against bowel cancer. Fibre cannot be completely digested. Different types of fibre provide varying numbers of calories but always fewer than simple carbohydrates (refined sugars).

After carbohydrates have been digested, they are broken down into simple sugars which are then stored as glycogen in the liver or muscle. Although it is metabolically possible to convert carbohydrate into fat, this rarely occurs.

Current dietary recommendations suggest that between 55 and 60 per cent of daily calorie intake should be consumed as carbohydrate, however the focus should be on complex carbohydrates which are a good

source of micronutrients and fibre. It is recommended that simple carbohydrates should be no more than about 10 per cent of your calorie intake, particularly if you are trying to lose weight.

Diets very low in carbohydrates can be dangerous, possibly leading to mineral imbalances, hypoglycaemia and interference with the efficiency of the body's metabolism.

FATS AND YOUR WEIGHT

In any diet which aims to control weight, fats should be kept to a minimum. Most nutritionists recommend that fat should comprise no more than 30 to 35 per cent of the daily intake with a maximum of 10 per cent of this coming from saturated fats.

Fats are made up of fatty acid molecules and the combination of these molecules determines whether a particular kind of fat is saturated, monounsaturated or polyunsaturated. Some essential fatty acids (EFAs) are just that – essential for many bodily functions – so it is important to include a small amount of fat in your diet. If you exclude all the visible fat from your diet there is still likely to be enough invisible fat contained within the food you eat to prevent EFA deficiencies – unless you are following a very strict diet.

Polyunsaturated fats (found in fish and vegetable oils) are rich sources of EFAs. Monounsaturated fats (found in nuts and olive oil) help to control the level of cholesterol in your body. Saturated fats, found in meats and dairy products, do not have these essential benefits and so should be cut out of the diet as far as possible. Another type of fat, trans-fatty acid, is a processed fat found in margarines and foods such as cakes and biscuits. Trans-fatty acids have been linked both to coronary heart disease and cancer and should therefore be avoided as far as possible.

Any extra fat that you eat above your basic energy requirements will be stored on your body as fat. The only way to get rid of it after that is to decrease the calories that you eat and increase the calories that you burn by doing more regular exercise. The message is clear – keep all fats to a minimum, making sure that those you eat are 'good' fats (poly and monounsaturated) not 'bad' fats (saturated and trans-fatty acids). Always check the labels on food packaging

BURNING OFF CALORIES: *Tennis*

This competitive but social game can be played with one partner (singles) or in a group of four (doubles). It improves lower body strength and endurance while demanding muscle coordination.

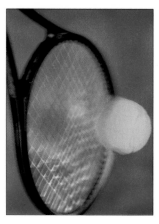

MUSCLE GROUPS BENEFITING
The lower torso and legs will benefit the most. The upper torso, shoulders and arms are stretched during strokes.

EQUIPMENT
Shorts and T-shirt. Supportive trainers are advisable.

CALORIES BURNT
Singles: about 7 calories per minute, (420 per hour). Doubles: about 6 calories per minute (360 per hour).

PLANNING YOUR MEALS TO GAIN WEIGHT

If you are 15 per cent or more below your expected weight range, and feel unduly fatigued, frequently chilly or, in the case of women, have missed three or more consecutive periods, you ought to consult your doctor as to whether you need to gain weight. In order to safely regain weight, your diet should follow basic healthy eating principles. Just as dramatic weight loss should be avoided, so should dramatic weight gain. The aim should be a gradual, steady increase. A sensible daily calorie intake for weight gain would be 3000 calories.

Follow a diet high in carbohydrate with modest amounts of fat and protein. Eat three main meals a day every day and drink lots of fruit juice and milk.

Increasing and maintaining weight levels is difficult without regular physical exercise. Muscles are more dense than fat, so muscle-building exercise is the best for weight gain. Your appetite may diminish when you start training but will increase again after a few days.

SAMPLE DAILY MENU FOR WEIGHT GAIN
The menu shown here provides a day's balanced diet following healthy eating rules and supplying a total intake of 3196 calories. It includes several rich sources of protein and carbohydrate, but is not too high in fat.

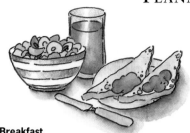

Breakfast
50 g (1¾ oz) cornflakes with dried fruit topping and 200 ml (7 fl oz) semi-skimmed milk; two slices of toast with jam and 2 tsp polyunsaturated margarine; 200 ml (6.8 fl oz) fresh orange juice = 736 calories

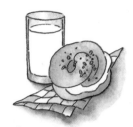

Mid morning snack
Bagel with 25 g (1oz) cream cheese and 225 ml (8 fl oz) semi-skimmed milk = 392 calories

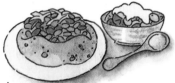

Lunch
Jacket potato with 250 g (9 oz) baked beans and grated cheddar cheese topping; 125 g (4½ oz) fruit salad with 125 g (4½ oz) custard made with semi-skimmed milk = 790 calories

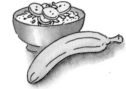

Afternoon snack
125 g (4½ oz) bowl of low-fat rice pudding and one sliced banana = 214 calories

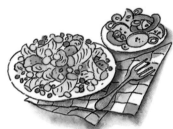

Dinner
Seafood pasta with 250 g (9 oz) boiled pasta, 90 g (3¼ oz) canned tuna in brine, 85 g (3 oz) peas, 90 g (3¼ oz) sweetcorn, 200 g (7 oz) tinned tomatoes, mixed herbs; salad with lettuce, tomatoes, cucumber, spring onions, cress, red and green peppers, olive oil and balsamic vinegar dressing = 682 calories

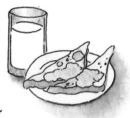

Supper
Two slices of toast with 25 g (1 oz) peanut butter and 225 ml (8 fl oz) warm semi-skimmed milk = 382 calories

to determine what kind of fats and how many are contained in the food. New synthetic fats are being developed which have fewer calories than other fats (natural fat provides nine calories per gram, more than twice as much by weight as protein or carbohydrate). The best known is Olestra (see page 74) which is now used in some snacks, such as crisps, in the United States.

VITAMINS AND MINERALS AND WEIGHT

Amidst concerns about counting calories it is easy to forget about vitamins and minerals, but these are essential to maintain good health while losing weight. The less food you eat the more care you need to take to ensure you eat foods with a high nutrient density – that is vitamins and minerals. Try to avoid foods, such as sugar, which contribute a lot of calories but do not deliver micronutrients. If you are in any doubt, consult a doctor or dietitian for advice. They may advise taking a multivitamin and mineral supplement.

Diets which are very high in fibre can sometimes interfere with the absorption of vitamins and minerals. Also, if you are very underweight, you could be missing out on many vitamins and minerals, putting your health at risk (see page 51).

Finally, a healthy body is more likely to maintain a healthy weight because bodily functions will be more efficient, so getting your essential nutrients will help you in your weight-control programme.

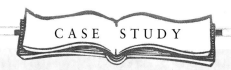

The Empty Calorie Eater

Many people who are overweight may not eat more food than people who are slim, but they eat the wrong types of foods – foods that are high in fat and sugar and low in fibre make up an empty calorie diet. This type of diet contains very little wholegrain cereals, fruits and vegetables and therefore provides a lot of energy but very few essential vitamins and minerals.

Ted is a 66-year-old man who, since retiring, has put on an excessive amount of weight and is now unhealthily overweight. He has always been a little on the plump side, but had managed to keep his weight within reasonable limits by walking to work every day and participating in a varied social life with his workmates. However, he now finds that without his daily exercise and with a less structured day, he lounges about the house watching the television, reading the newspaper and snacking frequently. The combination of very little physical exercise, other than

walking down the road to the local shop, and excess weight is making him less mobile, and he is starting to find that he is short of breath a lot of the time. Ted is also eating all the wrong kinds of food. Apart from a reasonably balanced evening meal, he consumes foods that are high in calories and fat and low in essential vitamins, minerals and fibres. He generally has a very light breakfast, but then fills up on biscuits or crisps until lunchtime, when he has a fried meal with bacon or sausages. He rarely eats vegetables before dinner, other than deep-fried chips. Ted also drinks

about four cans of beer a day. His wife, Sheila, who would also like to lose weight, suggested that Ted should visit the doctor. After an initial consultation, the doctor referred Ted to a State Registered Dietitian for a more thorough dietary assessment. Ted was asked to record his food intake for one week so that the dietitian could analyse the results for calories, fat, protein, carbohydrate and alcohol content. After careful examination, the dietitian advised Ted to alter his diet and increase his level of physical activity by taking more frequent exercise.

LIFESTYLE
Having an unstructured day can lead to weight gain. People can easily become sedentary which slows down their metabolic rate so that even fewer calories are burnt and more are laid down as fat.

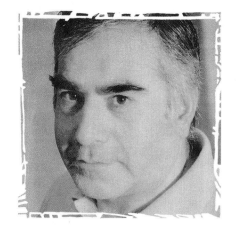

FOOD
Eating the wrong kinds of food will not only add unnecessary weight but will also contribute to other health problems such as high cholesterol.

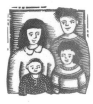

PARTNER/SPOUSE
It is much easier to lose weight if a close family member agrees to lose weight too.

EXERCISE
Being overweight can limit your physical abilities. This is a problem after retirement when you may wish to take up new activities.

RETIREMENT
Eating more and doing less exercise is a common cause of weight gain after stopping work.

WHAT SHOULD TED DO?

Ted should change his diet to cut down on fats and sugars and increase complex carbohydrates, fruits and vegetables. He should replace his usual breakfast of white toast and butter with wholewheat cereal or porridge, using low-fat milk and very little sugar or an artificial sweetener. This will fill him up more. He should also use low-fat milk in tea and coffee.

For lunches Ted should replace the fried foods with salads, lean meats or fish and low-fat dairy products. For snacks or dessert he should eat fruits, sorbets or low-fat yoghurt and not his accustomed crisps, chocolate bar or slice of cake. For his main meals Ted should eat plenty of vegetables, with either pasta, rice or potato (not fried) for carbohydrates, and beans, chicken, fish or lean meat for protein.

Any weight-loss plan should aim to reduce alcohol intake and Ted should try to cut his beer intake to one can per day. He should also try to cut down on the hours spent watching television as this is when he snacks, and he should try to increase the time spent on more active pursuits. He should make an effort to incorporate some kind of regular exercise into his life, such as a daily 30 minute walk. Gardening would be another way of getting a bit more activity into his life.

Action Plan

PARTNER/SPOUSE
Discuss weight loss plans with Sheila as she also wants to lose weight. Work out shopping lists and prepare meals together.

RETIREMENT
Plan ways of making better use of free time on a daily basis. Include more physical activity. Try to do some moderate exercise every day.

FOOD
Change diet to reduce fatty and sugary foods. Eat more fruits, vegetables and complex carbohydrates. Experiment with new recipes.

LIFESTYLE
Make a list of achievable goals towards a healthier lifestyle that can be attained over the next few months, such as gradually cutting down on the hours spent watching television. Use the extra time to plan and do some exercise.

EXERCISE
Start an exercise programme. Choose enjoyable activities and try to exercise daily for at least 30 minutes.

HOW THINGS TURNED OUT FOR TED

Ted, with the help of his wife Sheila, changed his diet along the lines recommended by the dietitian. In time both he and Sheila came to enjoy their new way of eating and looked forward to preparing new and exciting meals together each evening.

As part of their healthier lifestyle, they made a point of walking every morning for 30 minutes to an hour in the local park. At the weekends they started going for longer, more varied walks out in the countryside, even joining a local rambling club.

Within about six months, Ted had lost 10 kg (22 lb) and Sheila had also lost weight. His mobility gradually improved with the regular exercise and he became less breathless. This meant that he was able to walk at a quicker pace and he began to enjoy his morning walks more than before. The pair are now very keen walkers and have taken a number of short holidays based around interesting walks. This gives them something to plan for and look forward to, providing physical and mental exercise.

Ted has more energy than he did prior to losing weight and is able to do the things he had planned for his retirement, such as redecorating the house, and growing many of the vegetables that now form a large part of their diet.

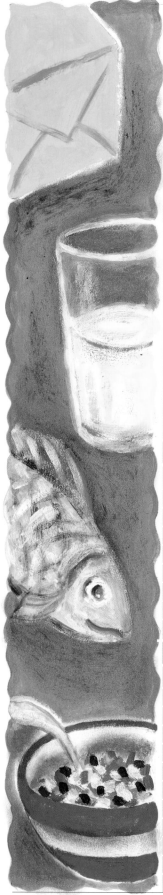

FOODS AND THEIR CALORIFIC VALUES

To control your diet properly you need accurate information about how healthy or unhealthy foods are. Studies have shown that people are poor judges of calorie and fat content. This chart will help you make better judgments about the food you eat. Bear in mind that the figure given for grams of fat per 100 g is not the same as percentage of fat, because it does not take into account the higher calorie content of fats. How to calculate the fat percentage is explained on page 73.

FOOD GROUP	CALORIES per 100 g (3½ oz)	FAT g per 100 g (3½ oz)	AVERAGE SERVING SIZE	CALORIES (per serving)	FAT (g per serving)
DAIRY PRODUCTS					
Brie	319	26.9	50 g/2 oz	160	13.5
Butter	737	82	25 g/1 oz	184	20.5
Cheddar cheese	412	34.4	50 g/2 oz	206	17.2
Cottage cheese	98	3.9	50 g/2 oz	49	2
Edam cheese	333	25.4	50 g/2 oz	166	12.7
Fruit yoghurt	90	0.7	150 g/5½ oz	135	1.1
Low-fat natural yoghurt	52	1	150 g/5½ oz	78	1.5
Low-fat spread	390	40.5	25 g/1 oz	97.5	10.1
Margarine	739	82	25 g/1 oz	187	20.5
Skimmed milk	33	0.1	1 glass, 200 ml/7 fl oz	66	0.2
Whole milk	66	3.9	1 glass, 200 ml/7 fl oz	132	7.8
MEAT AND FISH					
Beef, roasted topside	214	12	100 g/3½ oz	214	12
Chicken, roasted	216	14	115 g/4 oz	248	16.1
Lamb, roasted	266	17.9	100 g/3½ oz	266	17.9
Pork sausages, grilled	318	24.6	100 g/3½ oz	318	24.6
Turkey, roasted	171	6.5	115 g/4 oz	196.7	7.5
Cod, baked	96	1.2	100 g/3½ oz	96	1.2
Mackerel, fried	188	11.3	115 g/4 oz	216	12.9
Salmon, steamed	197	13	115 g/4 oz	226	14.9
Tuna, in brine	99	0.6	115 g/4 oz	114	0.7
CEREAL PRODUCTS					
Boiled rice	138	1.3	150 g/5½ oz	207	1.95
Cream crackers	440	16.3	2 biscuits, 14 g/½ oz	62	2.3
Lentils, red	100	0.4	100 g/3½ oz	100	0.4
Muesli	363	5.9	40 g/1½ oz	145	2.4
Popcorn (air popped)	388	3.8	15 g/½ oz	58	0.6
Puffed rice	369	0.9	40 g/1½ oz	148	0.4
Savoury rye biscuits	321	2.1	2 biscuits, 40 g/1½ oz	128	0.8
Savoury wheat biscuits	413	11.3	3 biscuits, 60 g/2¼ oz	248	2.8
Spaghetti	104	0.7	150 g/5½ oz	156	1.1
Tofu, steamed	73	4.2	100 g/3½ oz	73	4.2
White bread	235	1.9	2 slices, 70 g/2½ oz	165	1.33
Wholemeal bread	215	2.5	2 slices, 70 g/2½ oz	151	1.75

FOOD GROUP	CALORIES per 100 g (3½ oz)	FAT g per 100 g (3½ oz)	AVERAGE SERVING SIZE	CALORIES (per serving)	FAT (g per serving)
FRUITS AND VEGETABLES					
Apples, eating	45	0.1	115 g/4 oz	52	0.1
Bananas	95	0.3	130 g/4½ oz	124	0.39
Nectarines	40	0.1	130 g/4½ oz	52	0.1
Oranges	37	0.1	100 g/3½ oz	37	0.1
Peaches	33	0.1	140 g/5 oz	46	0.1
Baked beans	84	0.6	100 g/3½ oz	84	0.6
Broccoli, boiled	24	0.8	50 g/2 oz	12	0.4
Carrots, boiled	24	0.4	100 g/3½ oz	24	0.4
Celery, raw	7	0.2	50 g/2 oz	3.5	0.1
Cucumbers	10	0.1	50 g/2 oz	5	0.05
Green peppers, raw	15	0.3	50 g/2 oz	7.5	0.15
Lettuce	14	0.5	50 g/2 oz	7	0.25
Mushrooms, fried	157	16.2	50 g/2 oz	79	8.1
Potatoes, baked	136	0.2	150 g/5½ oz	204	1.3
Potatoes, boiled	72	0.1	150 g/5½ oz	108	0.15
Potatoes, chipped	239	12.4	150 g/5½ oz	359	18.6
Potatoes, mashed	104	4.3	150 g/5½ oz	156	6.5
Tomatoes	17	0.3	60 g/2¼ oz	10	0.2
DRINKS					
Beer (ales and bitters)	32	Negligible	600 ml/1 pint	192	Negligible
Cola	39	Nil	1 can, 330 ml/11 fl oz	129	Nil
Grapefruit juice	33	0.1	1 glass, 330 ml/11 fl oz	109	0.33
Gin	222	Nil	1 unit, 25 ml/¾ fl oz	55	Nil
Lager	29	Negligible	600 ml/1 pint	274	Negligible
Lemonade	21	Nil	1 can, 330 ml/11 fl oz	69	Nil
Mineral water	Nil	Nil	1 can, 330 ml/11 fl oz	Nil	Nil
Red wine	68	Nil	1 glass, 125 ml/4 fl oz	85	Nil
White wine, dry	66	Nil	1 glass, 125 ml/4 fl oz	82	Nil
White wine, sweet	94	Nil	1 glass, 125 ml/4 fl oz	117	Nil
SNACKS					
Chocolate, milk	529	30.3	25 g/1 oz	132	7.6
Crisps	546	37.6	Regular bag, 30 g/1⅛ oz	164	11.3
Digestive biscuits	471	20.9	2 biscuits, 30 g/1⅛ oz	141	6.3
Low fat crisps	483	21.5	Medium bag, 40 g/1½ oz	193	8.6
Peanuts, roasted	602	53	Medium bag, 40 g/1½ oz	241	21.2
CONDIMENTS					
Mustard, English	226	14.4	1 tsp	11	0.7
Olive oil	899	99.9	1 tbsp	99	11
Salad cream	348	31	1 tbsp	70	6.2
Tomato ketchup	98	Negligible	1 tbsp	15	Negligible
Vegetable oil	899	99.9	1 tbsp	99	11

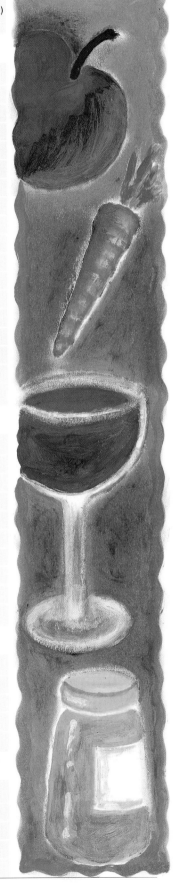

The Obesity Dietitian

Dietitians provide nutritional advice to people with a range of ailments where changes in diet can help to improve their health. Some dietitians (often called obesity dietitians) specialise in helping people lose weight because their weight is a health problem in itself.

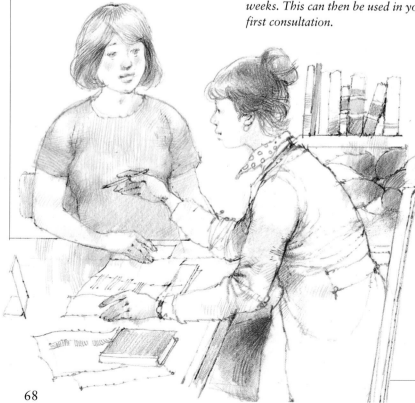

WEIGHTY MATTERS
Scales are an important part of the dietitian's armoury, essential for charting the patient's overall progress – but they should not be over-used or over-relied upon. To be healthy, weight loss should be gradual and slow, and lifestyle changes are more important than shedding pounds quickly.

Dietitians recognise that there are many different reasons why people are overweight. As therapists, they try to treat people as individuals, encouraging them to discuss the problem before giving out advice. As well as dietary recommendations, dietitians may also spend some time talking about positive lifestyle changes that can help a person to achieve an acceptable weight and then maintain it at that level.

HELPING THE DIETITIAN
It will help the dietitian to have a detailed breakdown of exactly what you eat. To make sure you remember everything, keep a diary of all the food and drinks you consume for a few weeks. This can then be used in your first consultation.

What sort of training do obesity dietitians have?
All dietitians have a degree, usually in nutrition and dietetics, and undergo additional training to become State Registered Dietitians. Their degree training covers the treatment of obesity in depth, and they may also have attended special training sessions organised by hospitals and research units.

What questions might a dietitian ask on the first visit?
Overweight patients who are referred to a dietitian because they wish to lose weight usually have other health problems as well. The dietitian will want to know their medical history, their previous experience with weight-reducing diets and if there is a history of obesity in their family. He or she will then assess the patient's current food intake and eating pattern throughout the day. For example, do they normally have breakfast, are meal times regular or do they eat sporadically? Finally, the dietitian may want to discuss in detail why they wish to lose weight. This might seem like an unnecessary question, but it can help establish the strength of the patient's motivation.

What dietary advice is given to overweight patients?
Dietary advice is carefully tailored to individual patient's needs, so it can vary tremendously, depending upon the patient's current food intake, lifestyle, the amount of weight that has to be lost, and whether the

patient has any other medical condition to take into account. Generally speaking, however, patients are encouraged to make gradual changes to their diet, incorporating more fruits, vegetables and whole grain cereals and reducing the proportion of foods that contain a lot of fat and sugar, such as cakes, biscuits, crisps and chocolate. Most dietitians do not ask patients to count calories, but instead encourage people to concentrate on making healthier food choices throughout their diet which they and their family can enjoy. In this way the 'diet' gradually becomes part of the patient's usual lifestyle.

Where do dietitians see their patients?

Dietitians work in hospital out-patient clinics, GP clinics or community centres. Patients may be seen either as individuals or in groups. For example, they may give talks to groups of patients attending a coronary rehabilitation class, or at education sessions organised for patients with diabetes. Many dietitians now see patients in GP surgeries, usually on an individual basis, which allows them to give more one-to-one attention.

How many appointments do patients usually have?

This depends very much on the nature of the weight problem. Some patients may be seen regularly, once a week or fortnight for an indefinite period of time if the causes of their weight problem are complex and they are benefiting from a lot of support. Alternatively, after the initial assessment and one follow-up appointment, you may be referred back to your GP or practice nurse so that they can monitor your progress, following the dietitian's advice.

Dietitians spend much of their time training practice nurses in how to help overweight and obese patients and these nurses are usually very good at offering long-term support and practical advice.

Are there any special techniques that dietitians use?

Yes, many dietitians use what are called behavioural therapy techniques to help their patients gain greater control over their eating habits. This is not as complicated as it sounds and simply involves working out some basic rules to help people eat when they are hungry and not for emotional reasons. For example, if you discuss with a dietitian that you feel a constant urge to snack, you may be advised to restrict your eating to one room in the house; for example, to the kitchen or dining room. In this way when you are sitting in the lounge or the bedroom you are less likely to be thinking about food since it is not a place where you ever eat. Similarly, you may be recommended not to eat while you are doing any other activity, for example, watching television. This is because with time there is the danger that your mind will connect the activities and eventually every time you sit down to watch television you will feel like having something to eat, whether you are hungry or not. A patient who requires further behavioural therapy may be referred to a psychologist for more specialised treatment.

Do dietitians work with other health professionals?

A dietitian will work closely with your GP or hospital doctor in order to understand fully any other medical problems you may have. Some dietitians work with psychologists (see above) in the treatment of obesity. For patients with specific eating disorders the psychologist may use cognitive therapy (see pages 40–41) to examine the cause of the disorder in depth and discuss potential solutions. Other dietitians work with exercise specialists, who can help to focus on diet and exercise combined to achieve the best long-term results.

WHAT YOU CAN DO AT HOME

If you have a tendency to be obsessed with food and find it difficult to keep to three meals a day without snacking in between, the following tips may help to put some routine back into your eating habits. This can be the start of regaining control over your weight.

▶ *Don't eat on the move or while watching TV. Always sit down to eat, and try to relax.*

▶ *Serve your meal on a medium-sized plate, not a large one. This will make the portion look larger.*

▶ *Immediately after serving yourself, wrap up any leftovers and put them in the refrigerator.*

▶ *Include planned healthy snacks in your diet – a piece of fruit, a low-fat yoghurt or something left over from dinner.*

TIMING YOUR MEALS

Eat your meals at the same time each day. You will find that your body quickly adjusts to more regular eating habits and you will feel less inclined to eat between meals.

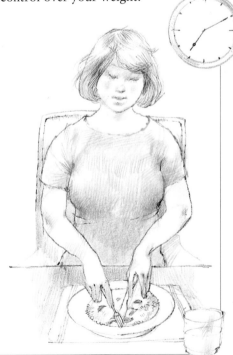

DRINKS AND WEIGHT CONTROL

There are various myths concerning how water, fruit juices, caffeinated drinks and alcohol can affect weight loss. The truth about which are beneficial to your health is actually very simple.

A high fluid intake is vital in order for your body to function properly – water plays a part in nearly all the body's functions. For this reason it is essential to keep up your fluid intake even when dieting. However, some drinks have quite a high calorie content so it is also important to choose low-calorie or calorie-free drinks.

WATER AND DIETING

Many overweight people believe that some of their excess weight is due to water retention and wonder if they should reduce their intake of water. They may well be retaining water, since obesity makes it more difficult for the body to return blood to the heart, and so water retention (or oedema) occurs. But drinking less water or taking diuretics is not the answer. Diuretic pills should be avoided, except under strict medical supervision, as they can lead to dehydration and any weight loss will be temporary. They can also cause the loss of essential nutrients from the body. Weight loss as a result of consuming fewer calories and exercising more will improve circulation of the blood and relieve oedema. Whether you are trying to lose weight or not you should aim to drink the equivalent of six to eight glasses of water a day.

CALORIE CONTENT OF SOME SOFT DRINKS

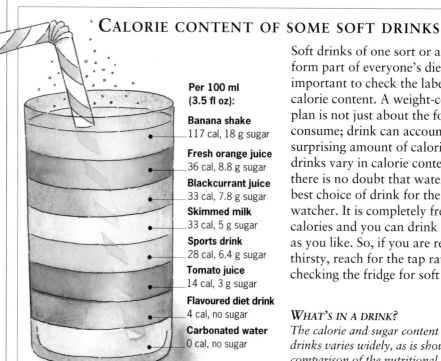

Per 100 ml (3.5 fl oz):

Banana shake
117 cal, 18 g sugar

Fresh orange juice
36 cal, 8.8 g sugar

Blackcurrant juice
33 cal, 7.8 g sugar

Skimmed milk
33 cal, 5 g sugar

Sports drink
28 cal, 6.4 g sugar

Tomato juice
14 cal, 3 g sugar

Flavoured diet drink
4 cal, no sugar

Carbonated water
0 cal, no sugar

Soft drinks of one sort or another form part of everyone's diet but it is important to check the labels for calorie content. A weight-control plan is not just about the food you consume; drink can account for a surprising amount of calories. Diet drinks vary in calorie content, and there is no doubt that water is the best choice of drink for the weight-watcher. It is completely free of calories and you can drink as much as you like. So, if you are really thirsty, reach for the tap rather than checking the fridge for soft drinks.

WHAT'S IN A DRINK?
The calorie and sugar content of soft drinks varies widely, as is shown in this comparison of the nutritional content of eight popular drinks.

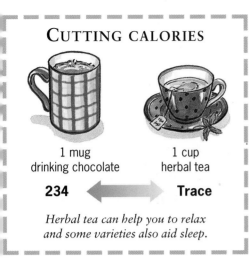
Caffeinated drinks

There is no calorific difference between caffeinated drinks and their decaffeinated alternatives. Regular coffee obviously contains caffeine, but caffeine is also added to colas, and a similar compound to caffeine, called theophylline, is present in tea. Caffeine stimulates the metabolic rate and therefore can, in theory, help to burn up calories, but this effect is too small to significantly affect weight loss. Excess caffeine is thought to be addictive and unhealthy. Side effects include insomnia, hyperactivity in children, and irritability.

Herbal teas provide a healthy alternative, and are virtually calorie free when drunk without milk or sugar.

Alcohol and your weight

Alcohol is high in calories and should be minimised as part of your weight-control programme. Units of alcohol are not an accurate guide to the calorific content of a drink – 1 g of pure alcohol contains 7 calories. A popular misconception is that pilsner lagers are lower in calories because 'more of the sugar is turned to alcohol'. However, since 1 g of sugar containing 4 calories is converted to 1 g of alcohol which contains 7 calories, a pilsner lager actually contains more calories than an ordinary lager.

In addition, alcohol can stimulate your appetite. People who are trying to gain weight are often advised to have an alcoholic drink before a meal. If you are trying to lose weight it is better to avoid alcohol altogether. The influence of alcohol can destroy your will-power and the intention to limit intake to just one or two drinks can quickly disappear. You may also be tempted to eat a high-fat snack which you might otherwise have resisted.

If you are used to drinking alcohol regularly and cannot give it up, allow yourself one drink before dinner or later in the evening as part of your whole diet plan. Try to stick to small measures and make sure that you can keep to a limited amount – don't let one drink slip into two. See page 53 for tips on how to limit alcohol during a weight-control plan.

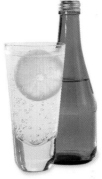

BON APERITIF!
Some people find that drinking carbonated water before a meal fills them up and as a consequence they eat less during the meal.

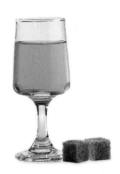

WHICH IS THE LESSER OF TWO EVILS?
When people think of a weight-loss plan, they automatically think of cutting back on fat and sugar. Often alcohol is overlooked and some people even congratulate themselves for missing a meal because they were at the pub with colleagues. In fact, alcohol contains almost twice as many calories per gram as sugar, so that liquid lunch could cost you your waistline.

FRUIT OR FRUIT JUICE?

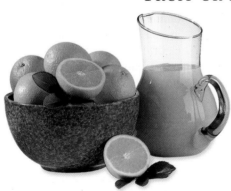

WHAT IS THE DIFFERENCE?
1 litre (1¾ pints) of unsweetened orange juice provides about 360 calories, 88 g sugar, 0.4 g fibre and 390 mg vitamin C. Five large oranges would weigh about the same, and when eaten without peel, supply 370 calories, 85 g sugar, 17 g fibre and 540 mg vitamin C.

Fruit juices contain useful amounts of vitamin C for people who do not eat much fruit or vegetables, such as young children and teenagers. However, if you receive enough vitamin C from whole fruit and vegetables, fruit juice can simply act as a source of calories. It is easy to consume a large amount without realising how many calories you are consuming when drinking orange juice for thirst. Juices are also relatively low in fibre because this is retained in the pulp of the fruit, which is discarded during juice extraction. When buying fruit juices, always choose unsweetened varieties and avoid those with additives or those which are simply high-sugar soft drinks based on juice concentrate.

THE FACTS ABOUT 'HEALTH FOODS'

The label 'health food' may sometimes be misleading. Unintentionally or otherwise, manufacturers add to the confusion when using the terms 'low-fat' and 'low-calorie'.

Advertising for some health foods implies that their consumption will confer health benefits on the consumer. Claims may be generalised or specifically related to a certain disease or problem. Many claims made for 'health foods' are very difficult to substantiate. Some products that claim to be 'natural' can have undesirable effects in large quantities, such as those that contain strong herbs.

An example of a product that is advertised as 'natural', but which may not offer any greater or lesser health benefits compared to its 'unnatural' alternative is bottled water (compared with tap water). Tap water is not pure, but then neither is bottled water. Some bottled waters may contain high levels of minerals which are unsuitable for children and people with hypertension. Moreover, many bottled mineral waters are flavoured and can contain high levels of sugar making them bad news for a weight-control plan.

In the same way that labelling of 'health' foods can be misleading, so can claims for 'natural' or 'healthy' aids to slimming. There are no specific slimming products that work long-term without changing your diet and lifestyle. Many of them act as diuretics and make you lose water not fat.

FOOD PACKAGING – BEHIND THE IMAGE

Tape measures will catch your eye and are a marketing ploy to make sure you instantly recognise this as a product that 'can be used as part of a calorie controlled diet'

Nutritional labels will reveal the truth about calorie content and any additives which may not match the healthy image

TRICKS OF THE TRADE
Packaging can be used to convey a 'healthy' image. Words such as 'slimline' and 'low-fat' in tall, slim letters will further enhance the message.

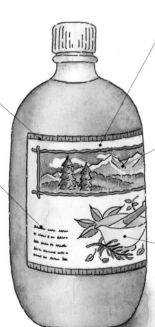

Pale colours are used to to give the product a clean, almost clinical look. This may be intended to give the impression that it is 'medically' good for you

Mountain scenery is often pictured to give the impression that the product is so natural that it has an affinity with nature itself

Imagery such as a pestle and mortar surrounded by herbs may be used to give the impression that the product is made with natural ingredients

It is important to read between the lines when shopping to ensure that you are not taken in by packaging gimmicks and marketing ploys. There are many tricks that manufacturers use to convince you that their product should be a regular part of your diet. The images presented can be misleading so you should always read the contents label carefully. Sometimes because the product is fat-free or low in sugar, other additives may be included. With a little experience, you will soon discover which products are valid for inclusion in your weight-control plan and can really help to make your daily diet more healthy.

Others contain stimulants to increase your metabolism which can be dangerous with long-term usage. If you really want to lose weight or maintain a healthy weight, you will have to change your eating and exercise habits – unfortunately there is no miracle answer in a bottle.

VALUE OF 'HEALTHY FOODS'

The nutritional and calorific value of health foods is as variable as all other foods. The important message is that 'health foods' do not necessarily contain more nutritional value or fewer calories compared with foods that are not labelled as 'health foods'. Some foods are naturally low in fat and therefore a good choice for a weight-control plan. These include fruits and vegetables, and many packaged products such as yoghurt, breakfast cereals and jams.

'Low-fat' health foods

Many foods are labelled as reduced fat, low-fat, lower fat, very low fat, light, or lite. This labelling actually means very little as it does not tell you about the absolute fat or calorie content of the food, or whether it is lower in fat than the alternatives. The differences between low-fat versions of some products, including yoghurt, cheese and biscuits, compared to their regular counterparts is not always significant. To find out what the real difference is you must look at the nutritional content on the label, and assess for yourself whether it is a worthwhile substitution. This may seem tedious at first but you will soon learn which foods to select.

Calculating fat content

The fat content of your total daily calorie intake should be no more than 30 to 35 per cent. There is a simple formula you can use to calculate the percentage of fat in a food item. Most packaged food now lists the weight of fat per 100 grams of the food but this does not give you the percentage of fat in the food because it does not take into account the number of calories and the fact that the nutritional components of the food have different calorie counts.

To calculate fat content, multiply the amount of fat per 100 g by 9. Divide the result by the food item's calories per 100 g. Multiply this number by 100 and this is your answer. For example if a packet of low-calorie sandwiches contains 194 calories with 4.9 g of fat per 100 grams it is 22.7 per cent fat:

$$4.9 \times 9 = 44.1 \div 194 = 0.227$$
$$0.227 \times 100 = 22.7 \text{ per cent}$$

In order to keep your daily fat intake at around 30 to 35 per cent, try to avoid eating food with a fat formula more than this, and balance high and low-fat foods. You'll soon be able to spot low-fat items without having to use the formula.

'Low-cholesterol' foods

Foods labelled 'low cholesterol' or 'no cholesterol' can be misleading; in fact, it is not the cholesterol you eat that creates high blood cholesterol levels – it is the amount of saturated fat you eat. If you need to cut

Foods that make false claims

The United Kingdom Food Labelling Regulations (1994) make it an offence to claim that a food can prevent, treat or cure a human disease or change your weight. However, magazines can publish articles promoting a particular product as long as it is stated that they are presenting an opinion only. A number of so-called health foods are promoted in this way. The Trading Standards Office has the power to investigate health claims made about particular products and can prosecute if a claim is false. Misleading adverts can also be referred to the Advertising Standards Authority.

A COMPARISON OF SPREADS

Originally margarine was manufactured as a war-time substitute for butter but has now become a product in its own right and spawned many variants which can combine butter's taste with margarine's spreadability. This comparison shows the differences in the nutritional values of four different types of spreads.

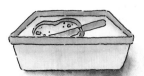

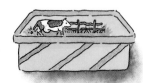

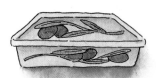

SPREADS THAT ARE VERY LOW IN FAT
Per 100 g: about 273 calories, 25g fat and negligible cholesterol.

BLENDS OF DAIRY PRODUCTS AND VEGETABLE OILS
Per 100 g: about 739 calories, 81.6 g fat and 225 mg cholesterol.

MARGARINES THAT ARE HIGH IN POLYUNSATURATES
Per 100 g: about 739 calories, 81.6g fat and 7 mg cholesterol.

SPREADS WITH AN OLIVE OIL BASE
Per 100 g: about 545 calories, 60 g fat, and negligible cholesterol.

WHICH SNACKS ARE HEALTHY?

There are lots of low-calorie, low-fat snacks that will leave you feeling guilt-free and satisfied. Keep your kitchen stocked with the foods listed below:

▶ *Bread with a low-fat topping such as tuna mixed with tomato*

▶ *Fresh salad with vinegar or lemon dressing*

▶ *Savoury biscuits (choose a low-fat variety) with cottage cheese*

▶ *Rice cakes*

▶ *Air-popped corn*

▶ *Breakfast cereal with skimmed milk*

▶ *Low-fat yoghurt with any fruit – try blending yoghurt and fruit for a delicious drink*

▶ *Fruit (fresh or tinned in natural juices)*

▶ *Low-sugar sorbet*

▶ *A handful of dried fruit such as raisins, apricots and figs*

A HEALTHY TREAT
Vegetables are low in fat and also have greater amounts of vitamins and minerals when eaten raw. Try sticks of carrot, celery and cucumber with a low-fat dip such as yoghurt or cottage cheese with herbs or chives.

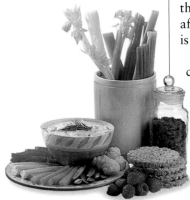

down your blood cholesterol levels you should avoid foods with a high content of saturated fats. And if you are watching your weight, you should cut down on all fats. The 'low cholesterol' or 'no cholesterol' labels do not mean that the product will help you lose weight. For example, substituting 'low cholesterol' margarine for butter will not lower your weight – they both contain the same amount of calories. Margarine, however, will make a difference to your health by lowering your risk of heart disease as it contains more unsaturated fat than butter.

Sugar variations

Although some types of sugars are regarded by consumers as being more healthy than others, all sugars contain the same amount of calories per weight. Therefore if you are trying to lose weight or maintain a healthy weight, you should cut down on all sugars, including brown sugar, honey and syrup.

Sugar substitutes

Some sugar substitutes such as mannitol, sorbitol, xylitol and hydrogenated glucose syrup contain almost the same amount of calories as sugar and so are not helpful in a weight-control diet. Others, however, including acesulfame K, aspartame and saccharin, contain virtually no calories. As part of a weight-loss programme, they are useful for sweetening foods and drinks and you could also choose products that use them instead of sugar. But instead of satisfying a sweet tooth with artificial sweeteners, it is more beneficial to change your eating habits to include a variety of healthy, low-sugar foods and naturally sweet foods like fruit.

Substitutes for 'naughty' foods

Some 'health foods' are presented as substitutes for so called 'naughty foods', giving the impression that eating them will not affect your weight-control programme. This is not always the case.

Carob, a popular substitute for chocolate, contains the same amount of calories. Likewise, dark and milk chocolate contain the same amount of calories and frozen yoghurt is no less fattening than ice-cream, unless it is a low-fat version. Sorbet is a better substitute for ice cream, though some varieties are high in sugar – so look for low-sugar brands.

OLESTRA

Olestra has recently been approved in the United States for use in snack foods and may arrive in Britain in the future. It tastes and cooks like real fat but won't cause weight gain because it cannot be absorbed by the body. All this sounds too good to be true but there are drawbacks – it can cause diarrhoea and abdominal cramps, if eaten in large quantities. Research also suggests that Olestra binds to the vitamins A, D, E and K and the carotenoids (antioxidants which protect against heart disease and cancer) and carries them with it through and out of the body. Although vitamins will be added to products made with Olestra, carotenoids will not. A sensible approach is to select naturally low-fat products where possible and only eat foods made with Olestra when there is no substitute.

It is possible, however, to substitute low-calorie foods for the high-calorie version without compromising on taste, by using low-fat, low-sugar and low-calorie products. Always check labels and compare brands to ensure you really are choosing a product that makes a difference. Compare total fat content, sugar content and calories per 100 g for similar products – if the difference is at least 20 per cent, it is probably worth trying.

It is also important to completely replace those foods in your diet that are particularly high in fat. Yoghurt is a useful substitute for cream, can be added to sauces to give a creamy texture and substituted for mayonnaise or butter on baked potatoes. Sour cream contains the same number of calories as ordinary cream but low-fat crème fraîche has fewer, and does not curdle when boiled.

Mayonnaise is extremely high in calories so for sandwiches try substituting pickles or mustards, which are tasty but low in fat. Try to get into the habit of having sandwiches without butter or margarine and instead use low-fat spreads and spread it very thinly. Avoid oily salad dressings – use different flavoured vinegars mixed with lemon juice instead or add low-fat yoghurt for a creamier dressing.

CHAPTER 5

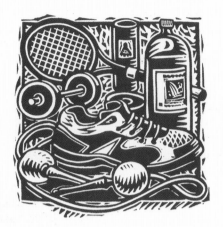

EXERCISE AND YOUR WEIGHT

Exercise, in some form, is a vital part of any weight-control programme. Combining careful management of your diet with regular exercise is, without doubt, the most successful way to reach and maintain your ideal weight. Exercise has the added benefit of increasing fitness and general well-being.

USING EXERCISE TO CONTROL WEIGHT

In the past, the emphasis in weight reduction has been on calorie restriction. Today, however, it is known that weight management is most successful when exercise and diet work hand-in-hand.

If you take in more energy (calories) through the food you eat than your body requires for general functioning, you will gain weight – the excess energy not used up by your body is converted to fat and stored. If your intake and output of energy are equal your weight will remain constant. The best long-term solution for weight loss, therefore, is to reduce your energy intake by adapting your diet and also increase your energy output by doing more exercise.

Dieting alone can be difficult to maintain. You may feel weak and lethargic if you reduce your intake too dramatically, and it may be difficult to maintain strict control over the food you eat. There is also clinical evidence to support the importance of exercise in weight control: one recent study in the United States, for example, followed the progress of two groups over a period of 12 weeks. One group followed a low calorie diet; the second group followed the same diet, but carried out an exercise programme at the same time. The second group were not only more successful at losing weight in the short term, they were also more successful at maintaining the weight loss. A follow up of the two groups after 24 weeks showed that the exercise group had on average regained only 0.4 kg (14 oz) in weight compared with the diet-only group's average weight regain of 1.8 kg (4 lb).

EXERCISE AND WEIGHT LOSS

The body uses energy just to keep itself alive: breathing, making the heart beat, maintaining organ functions and producing heat all call on energy converted by the body from the food you eat. During exercise, additional demands are placed on the body's supply of energy. Different types of physical activity make different energy demands – strenuous exercise like swimming continuously for 20 minutes will always burn more energy than, for example, walking. But you can still achieve a significant weight loss with only moderate exercise if this is done on a daily basis.

MUSCLE VERSUS FAT

Muscle and fat cells have a different cellular structure and have specific functions. Fats, or lipids, are stored as adipose tissue just beneath the skin and around various internal organs and serve as a concentrated

THE HIDDEN FAT IN YOUR MUSCLES

Many people do not realise that considerable deposits of fat can be stored around muscle fibres. However, regular aerobic exercise can improve the condition of the muscles, increasing the number of capillaries running through them. This improves the supply of blood carrying oxygen to the muscles. The size and number of mitochondria enzymes (which produce energy) within each individual muscle cell also increases, so that the muscle is able to function much more efficiently.

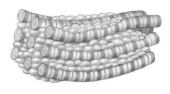

UNEXERCISED MUSCLE
The fibres of unexercised muscle are surrounded by fat deposits and the muscle itself is smaller and less oxygenated than exercised muscle.

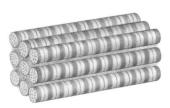

EXERCISED MUSCLE
Toned muscle becomes lean and increases in density, with more and larger capillaries and aerobic enzymes which promote more efficient energy production.

source of energy for the body. Adipose tissue makes up a larger portion of the total body weight of women than of men (about 20 to 25 per cent of total body weight, compared to 15 to 20 per cent for a man). This is principally to ensure that women have adequate energy stores for reproduction.

Muscle cells are long and slender in structure compared with round fat cells, and are capable of contraction and relaxation to create movement. There are three types of muscles: skeletal, smooth, and cardiac. Skeletal muscles are by far the largest group in the body. These muscles are under the body's conscious control; they are activated by the brain to perform various functions, like taking a step, and account for 40 to 45 per cent of total body weight. Smooth and

cardiac muscles are not under conscious control: they regulate the action of internal organs such as the bowel and the heart.

How muscles affect weight

Muscle cells weigh up to three times more than fat cells, which is why men generally weigh more than women height for height: more of their total body weight consists of muscle. But it takes more energy (calories) to fuel a muscle cell than a fat cell. Regular exercise will increase the bulkiness of muscles and their demand for fuel. In response, your metabolic rate will increase to provide the extra energy needed, by burning more calories, helping you to lose weight. A diet-only weight-loss plan can produce unwanted effects on your metabolic rate. About 25

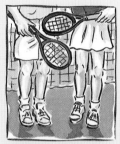

QUICK FITNESS TIP
Try to avoid planning your social occasions around eating out. Instead, invite your friends to play sport or go for a country walk.

COMBINING DIET AND EXERCISE

On a diet-only weight-loss programme, you will have to reduce your calorie intake much more significantly in order to lose weight than if you also had an exercise regime. Exercise both burns up calories directly and increases your metabolic rate. Below is a comparison of a day in the life of two different women who both weigh 10 stone (63.5 kg). Justine is moderately active, and so requires about 2500 calories per day to maintain her weight. In practice, her combination of exercise and

careful eating means that her calorie intake is less than this, and she will lose weight. Katie is quite sedentary during the week (but more active at weekends), and needs about 2000 calories per day. As her calorie intake is much higher she will gain weight unless she makes some lifestyle changes. She also eats far more fat than Justine, and studies show that the amount of fat in the diet is at least as important as the number of calories in determining weight gain and fat deposition.

JUSTINE'S DAY			
FOOD INTAKE	KCAL (FAT)	EXERCISE/ LIFESTYLE	KCALS BURNT
Breakfast – bran flakes, bagel with low fat spread, coffee (milk and sugar)	440 (16 g)	20 min brisk walk to bus	100
2 chocolate chip cookies	97 (5 g)		
Lunch – tuna (in brine) and salad sandwich, low-fat yoghurt, coffee	369 (3.2 g)	30 min brisk walk at lunch	150
Snack – dried currants	267 (0.4 g)	20 min brisk walk home	100
Dinner – roast chicken (without skin), baked potato, carrot, broccoli and trifle (without cream), fruit juice	800 (22 g)		
Snack – banana	95 (0.3 g)		
Bedtime drink – herbal tea	2		
TOTAL	2070 (46.9g)		350

KATIE'S DAY			
FOOD INTAKE	KCAL (FAT)	EXERCISE/ LIFESTYLE	KCALS BURNT
Breakfast – croissant with butter and jam, coffee (milk and sugar)	342 (18 g)	10 min drive to work	16
Doughnut	235 (10 g)		
Lunch – tuna (in oil) and salad sandwich, creamy yoghurt, coffee	497 (13 g)	Has lunch at her desk	16
Snack – mixed nuts/raisins	481 (34 g)	10 min drive home	16
Dinner – roast chicken (with skin), baked potato, fried tomato, carrot, broccoli and trifle (with cream) and 2 glasses wine	1136 (48 g)		
Snack – chocolate bar	736 (34 g)		
Bedtime drink – cocoa	127 (4.3 g)		
TOTAL	3554 (161.3 g)		48

How to prevent dehydration during exercise

It is vital to keep up your fluid levels during exercise. Becoming dehydrated can affect your ability to use your muscles and can make you physically ill. During an hour's exercise you can lose 1 litre (1¾ pints) of fluid through sweat and in the form of water vapour you breathe out. Be especially careful to keep up your fluid intake when exercising in very hot weather, and always ensure you take a supply of water with you when doing any exercise at all, even going for a walk. High-energy means high-calorie so sports drinks are best avoided during a weight-loss plan – water is the best choice for efficient rehydration without adding calories.

per cent of the weight lost in a diet-only regime is lean muscle. This means that you will lower your metabolic rate as less and less energy is required, and so make it harder to lose weight. Because exercise tones your muscles, it can also improve your general appearance, which is ultimately what most weight-loss plans are trying to achieve.

Can muscle turn into fat?

Happily, this common fear is a biological impossibility because the cellular composition and functions of muscle and fat are very different (see page 76). If you have been carrying out an exercise programme for a long time and then stop, your muscles will 'waste' relatively quickly, losing their firmness and tone. This may lead to their looking like 'fat', but once exercise is resumed your muscles will return to their former tone.

Avoiding muscle over-enlargement

Muscles can hypertrophy (enlarge) as a result of excessive and constant demand – such as during load bearing or resistance exercise like body building and, to a lesser extent, weight lifting. It can also happen in other more general activities such as step aerobics if performed to excess. If muscle size increases but body fat levels have not decreased simultaneously (because you have increased your calorie intake), you might look larger as layers of fat rest over the

ENERGY FOR EXERCISE

To be truly effective, your exercise plan needs to be properly fuelled. Not enough or the wrong fuel can make you feel prematurely tired. If your diet contains the recommended level of carbohydrates (see page 60) you will be eating enough for most exercise needs. But strenuous or prolonged exercise may need an extra energy boost such as a banana, jacket potato, or some fruit eaten two hours before. Up to two hours after exercise the body's system of food breakdown into usable energy such as glycogen is at its most efficient so it is important to refuel with a healthy meal and not high-fat snacks and drinks. The latter cannot be efficiently or completely broken down and much will be stored as fat.

muscle and you would also weigh more. But remember that it is not so much weight you are trying to control but fat. Weight is easy to measure but it is not always an accurate guide to body fat.

Whatever activity you choose, you can safeguard yourself by introducing a range of exercises that concentrate on different muscles. This is called cross-training and will result in all-over muscle improvement. It has the added benefit that variation in activity is less likely to cause injury as a result of repetitive physical stress, and you are less likely to become bored by always following the same training routine.

THE BEST FUEL FOR EXERCISE

It is widely understood that energy stored in the body is 'burnt off' during exercise but what is the most efficient fuel for exercise? Two sources of energy are used by the body: carbohydrates (stored as glycogen) and fat. Prolonged and high-intensity exercise leads the body to draw on complex carbohydrates and fat for fuel. Carbohydrate is the form of energy that the body can use most effectively; studies have shown that increasing the amount of carbohydrate eaten in the days before a competition can increase an athlete's ability to perform sustained, intense exercise. Fat, however, does not improve performance in high intensity exercise and can even make performance worse.

BURNING OFF CALORIES: *Low-impact Aerobics*

Aerobics is a series of movements and exercises put to music. You can either attend a class, or exercise to a home video. It is an ideal way of improving your fitness level with a low risk of injury.

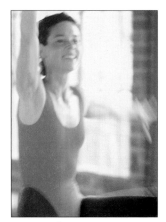

MUSCLE GROUPS BENEFITING
Some classes work all muscle groups while others, such as 'Legs, Bums and Tums', target specific areas.

EQUIPMENT
A good pair of training shoes that support your ankles. For women, a sports bra is also recommended.

CALORIES BURNT
8 calories are burnt per minute: that's 480 calories in an hour-long session.

Starting from scratch

There is some evidence that low-intensity exercise (aerobic activity in which breathing is easy, such as walking at a moderate pace) performed for long periods can burn up stored fat. Prolonged low-intensity exercise is a sensible way for overweight or very sedentary people to begin exercising. Every activity has a fat burning potential so try to include more physical effort in your daily life – for example, walk to the shops or part of the way to work, or decide to catch up on some gardening or housework. Begin a form of exercise that can be gradually increased to a moderate intensity as you become fitter. Short walks, for example, can be lengthened, the pace increased, and hills included as the weeks go by. Visits to your local swimming pool can be treated in the same way.

HOW EXERCISE AFFECTS METABOLISM

The amount of energy that your body uses at rest is determined by your metabolic rate (see page 29). If you can increase this you can lose weight more easily as your body calls upon more energy for everything from breathing to running. But it takes a long period of regular exercise to have this effect.

Although actually raising your metabolic rate can take a lot of hard work and a while to achieve, even light to moderate exercise can prevent the decrease in metabolic rate which would occur if you tried to lose weight by using a diet-only plan without increasing your activity levels.

EXERCISING AT THE RIGHT INTENSITY

Once you have achieved a reasonable level of fitness, learning to measure your heart rate will help you assess if your exercise routine is making your body work hard enough.

Your target heart rate zone is largely determined by your age and fitness levels. Find your maximum heart rate (beats per minute) by subtracting your age from 220. Multiply this figure by 0.55 and 0.85 to find a personal range at 55 per cent to 85 per cent of your maximum – this is the level you should aim for when you train. Your pulse during exercise should at least be up to the lower level but should not exceed the higher one. Take your pulse (see right) during and after activity to check that your training is both safe and effective – working at your maximum is not medically recommended. If the intensity is low – with a pulse of 55-65 per cent – the duration of the activity should be longer. If the intensity is greater – a pulse between 65-85 per cent – the duration can be shorter for the same effect. If your Body Mass Index is 30 or over (see page 25), if your resting heart rate is in the poor range, or if you have a medical condition, consult a doctor before setting heart rate targets.

Finding your average pulse rate

To find your average pulse rate, take your pulse (see below) on three separate mornings immediately after waking and calculate the average. Resting heart beats per minute are usually between 60 and 80 (lower for men, higher for women). Use the charts on the left to assess your pulse rate.

CHECKING YOUR PULSE RATE

To determine if your exercise routine is efficient, use your pulse rate as a guide. Your resting pulse reflects your true level of fitness and your pulse during exercise tells you how hard your body is working and can be a warning if the level is too high to be safe. Generally the lower your pulse rate the fitter you are.

RESTING PULSE RATE				
AGE	POOR	FAIR	GOOD	EXCELLENT
MEN				
20–29	86+	70–84	62–68	60 or less
30–39	86+	72–84	64–70	62 or less
40–49	90+	74–88	66–72	64 or less
50+	90+	76–88	68–74	66 or less
WOMEN				
20–29	96+	78–94	72–76	70 or less
30–39	98+	80–96	72–78	70 or less
40–49	100+	80–98	74–78	72 or less
50+	104+	84–102	76–82	74 or less

RECOVERY PULSE RATE AFTER 30 SECONDS				
AGE	POOR	FAIR	GOOD	EXCELLENT
MEN				
20–29	102+	86–100	76–84	74 or less
30–39	102+	88–100	80–86	78 or less
40–49	106+	90–104	82–88	80 or less
50+	106+	92–104	84–90	82 or less
WOMEN				
20–29	112+	94–110	88–92	86 or less
30–39	114+	96–112	88–94	86 or less
40–49	116+	96–114	90–94	88 or less
50+	118+	100–116	92–98	90 or less

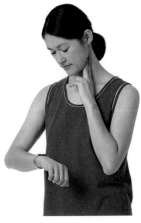

TAKING YOUR PULSE
Locate the carotid artery under the jaw using your fingers. Count the beats for 15 seconds and multiply by four – this is your minute reading.

THE RIGHT EXERCISE

Introducing more physical activity into your life needs to be planned to ensure that you choose the right type of exercise and the best routine to suit your age and lifestyle.

Warming-up correctly
A crucial part of every exercise session, warming up prepares your body for exercise by stimulating your cardiovascular system and preparing your muscles.

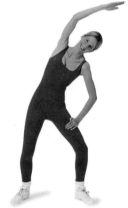

GENTLE STRETCHING
Stretch all the major muscle groups, keeping movements smooth, gentle and relaxed.

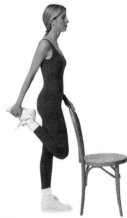

HOLDING THE STRETCH
For maximum benefit hold the stretch for 8–10 seconds, ensuring correct posture is maintained.

There are two types of exercise: aerobic and anaerobic. Aerobic exercise is any form of prolonged activity that can be performed continuously for at least 12 minutes and that uses oxygen to provide energy for the muscles. This includes brisk walking, jogging, cycling, swimming and aerobic dancing (body toning exercises set to music). The latter is either low-impact or high-impact: low-impact exercises tend to be slower and more controlled while high-impact exercise is more jarring on your body, involving jumps and running.

Anaerobic exercise consists of short, sharp bursts of strenuous activity such as weight lifting, sprinting or ballet. Different chemical reactions take place in the body to provide fuel for anaerobic exercise, and exercise cannot be maintained for long periods as the body's refuelling system is not as efficient. Aerobic exercise is therefore the best form of exercise both for efficient burning of calories and for your general health.

STARTING TO EXERCISE

It is important to be realistic when starting an exercise routine – you will only do more harm than good if you push yourself too hard at the beginning. Lack of fitness makes your heart less efficient at pumping blood to the muscles during exercise: they won't have enough oxygen to use as fuel and will tire more rapidly, and your reflexes will slow down. This increases the risk of injury.

If you are over 40, have an existing medical condition, have a BMI over 30, or if your resting heart rate is in the poor range (see page 79), it is sensible to have a check-up with your doctor before starting an exercise regime. Your doctor can check your blood pressure and heart rate and can advise you on a suitable level of exercise, and warn against particular forms of exercise which may be inappropriate.

When you first begin to exercise you may experience muscle aches but these will pass as the muscle group adjusts to being used. Warming up the muscles before exercise is important and will help to reduce the likelihood of aches and pains.

There are some warning signs from your body that should not be ignored. Fainting during exercise is a serious danger signal, as it suggests a reduced blood flow to the brain which could be due to a decrease in blood pressure or a sudden change in the rhythm of your heart. If you experience chest pains or extreme breathlessness, you should see your doctor as soon as possible.

Any increase in your level of activity should be implemented slowly. Guidelines issued by the British Health Education Authority recommend that adults should build up to 30 minutes or more of low to moderate intensity aerobic exercise on most, preferably all, days of the week. For example, you could begin with a ten-minute session twice a week, gradually increasing the length of time you perform the exercise and the number of sessions each week.

Low to moderate forms of aerobic exercise include walking, gentle swimming and gentle cycling. If activities such as

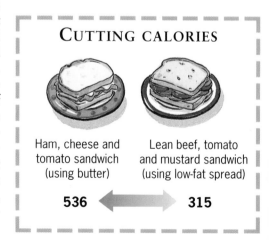

CUTTING CALORIES

Ham, cheese and tomato sandwich (using butter)

Lean beef, tomato and mustard sandwich (using low-fat spread)

536 ⬅➡ **315**

housework and gardening are sufficiently vigorous and prolonged to raise your heart rate, they would also count as reasonable forms of exercise. Older people may benefit from specially designed low-impact exercise classes held at local leisure centres and community halls. The key to success, however, is that the exercise is performed at least three times a week on a regular basis.

THE BEST TIME TO EXERCISE

Once you have begun your new exercise regime it is important that you maintain it, so arrange to exercise at times which fit most readily into your existing lifestyle. For example, if your job is demanding and stressful, an exercise break in the middle of the day can help relieve tension, clear your mind, and actually make you more effective in your job for the remainder of the day. There may be a gym near where you work where you could use the exercise bike for 20 minutes, or use the step machine. With little enough time to fit in both work and social activities, many people cannot even consider exercising in the evening. If your evenings are always busy, consider swimming in the morning before work. Many pools open early enough to allow this, and it can be a great way to start the day.

If you have a family, look at ways of making the evening a time for family exercise. Could you all go for a bike ride, for example, or go swimming in an indoor pool twice a week? Again, this will not only provide you with useful exercise; it will also be fun time spent with the family, and in addition will probably help to give you a good night's sleep. It is important that once you have established the most convenient time for you to exercise you go regularly.

RISKS OF OVER-EXERCISING

Over-exercising is potentially as harmful as under-exercising. Unless the body is given time to recover after each exercise session, the continuous wear can lead to muscle injuries such as strains or tears. Gentle, regular exercise, such as walking, can be performed several times a week but more strenuous exercise, such as a workout at the gym, should be followed by a rest day so that muscles can recover. Erratic bouts of exercise without proper warm up and cool down exercises can put unhealthy strain on the heart, particularly in older people.

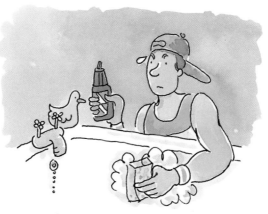

Excessive exercising can also cause more serious health problems. Strenuous exercise in very hot weather may lead to heat exhaustion. Symptoms include dizziness, nausea and cramps. In serious cases heat stroke can result which can be life threatening. To avoid heat exhaustion ensure you drink plenty of water before, during and after exercise. Wear light, comfortable clothing, and in very hot weather, consider exercising later in the evening.

Long-term strenuous exercise for women may also lead to amenorrhea (the cessation of menstruation), by reducing the level of hormones which control the menstrual cycle. If your weight drops substantially below the

continued on page 84

ELBOW GREASE
Housework can burn a surprising number of calories, especially if you put your back into it. Light housework, like dusting or hoovering, can burn up to 4 calories per minute. Vigorous activities, like scrubbing the bath or moving furniture, can burn between 5 and 7.5 calories per minute.

AEROBIC VERSUS ANAEROBIC EXERCISE

Aerobic exercise needs a steady supply of oxygen to the muscles. It improves cardiovascular fitness and uses up fat stores for energy. Anaerobic exercise is targeted to build muscle rather than improve fitness, and only burns carbohydrate stores, not fat. This type of exercise cannot be sustained for long periods – you can feel exhausted after just a minute or so – and the build-up of lactic acid, a by-product of the anaerobic reaction, can cause muscle pain and fatigue.

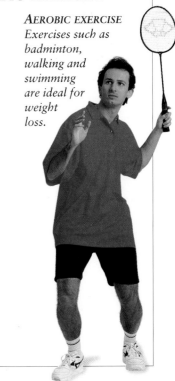

AEROBIC EXERCISE
Exercises such as badminton, walking and swimming are ideal for weight loss.

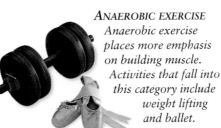

ANAEROBIC EXERCISE
Anaerobic exercise places more emphasis on building muscle. Activities that fall into this category include weight lifting and ballet.

Skipping

Skipping is one of the best forms of aerobic exercise. It burns off lots of calories, is easy and fun and can be done at home without expensive equipment. As a low impact exercise, it won't put your knees under stress, and will loosen up your shoulders.

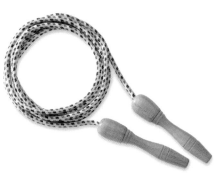

A COMPLETE WORK-OUT
Skipping is a low impact exercise as your feet generally stay close to the ground. It provides very effective all-round exercise, working your back and shoulders and improving the range of movement in your shoulder joints.

Many people don't exercise enough. Some find professionally run classes or gym membership too expensive or find it hard to attend classes regularly. Others may feel embarrassed about exercising in front of other people. But these shouldn't be reasons not to exercise:

the answer is to devise a simple routine that can be practised at home. Skipping is a useful exercise to increase your total physical fitness. It targets your calves, thighs and buttocks, and can easily be done at home – all you need is enough room to swing the rope.

WARMING UP AND COOLING DOWN

Begin all forms of exercise with some basic warm-up stretches like the ones shown here. These should last approximately 10 minutes. Use the same stretches to cool down after your exercise session.

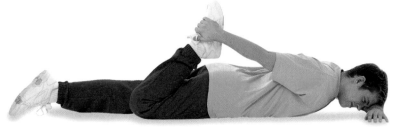

THIGH STRETCH
Lie face down with your stomach in and your hips pressed to the floor. Rest your forehead on your left arm, keeping your head in line with your spine. With knees together, bend your right knee, reaching

back with your right hand to pull your foot towards your buttocks. When you feel tension in the front of your thigh, hold the stretch for 8 to 10 seconds. Repeat with the other leg.

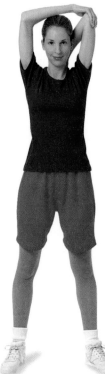

ARM STRETCH
Stand with your back straight, your stomach tucked in and your hips slightly tilted forward. Your feet should be about hip width apart, and your knees slightly bent. Raise your left arm and lower your hand behind your head, between your shoulder blades. Placing your right hand over your left elbow, ease your elbow towards the midline of your body. Keep your head upright and facing forward. Hold the stretch for 8 to 10 seconds. Repeat with the other arm.

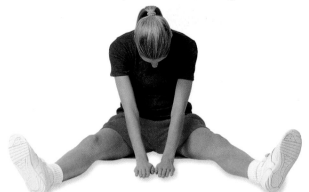

GROIN STRETCH
Sit with your back straight, legs apart and stomach pulled in. Start off with head up and hands on inner thighs. Bend

forward from hips and place hands flat on floor in front of you. Reach forward until you feel tension in the groin. Keep your toes pointing up.

BUYING THE RIGHT ROPE

The most important thing when buying a skipping rope is to ensure it is the right length. Also make sure to get a hard-wearing, heavy rope.

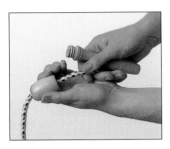

SHORTENING THE ROPE
It is usually possible to adjust the length if the rope is too long. Check before you buy.

MEASURING UP
Stand with both feet on the centre of the rope and pull up the ends. The handles should reach to your armpits. It is advisable to measure this with string first so that you get a long enough rope.

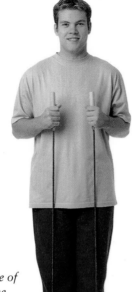

BUILDING UP A REGIME

Many people assume that because skipping is a popular game for children, it cannot be a strenuous exercise that adults can use. But in practice, skipping is a lot harder than it looks.

A regular skipping programme will help you to develop your fitness coordination and agility, and also makes an excellent addition to a cross-training programme. This is where a variety of aerobic and resistance activities – such as skipping and weight lifting – are combined to create a complete cardiovascular workout to achieve all-round fitness.

INTRODUCING A ROUTINE
If you have not skipped for some time, you may find a normal training level too hard. To build up a routine, skip initially for 2 minutes, or if this is too much, for 30–40 skips, and then rest for 30 seconds. Repeat twice. At each subsequent session reduce the rest intervals by 5 seconds a time until you have eliminated them.

STARTING A REGIME
You should now be ready to begin a formal training regime but this should still be introduced gradually. Start with a 3 minute skipping session once a week; then graduate to a 4 minute session twice a week; then a 5 minute session twice a week, building up over ten sessions to three 20 minute sessions a week.

SKIPPING FOR BEGINNERS

Wearing loose, comfortable clothing and training shoes, begin to skip. Try to keep your shoulders relaxed and your upper arms close to your body. Use your wrists, not your whole arms, to turn the rope and try to keep them as low as possible. Keep your back straight and your stomach pulled in.

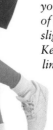

ROCKING SKIP
This is the easiest type of skipping, and because you are half running rather than jumping, it does not require as much energy. Step with the same foot leading, then try alternating the leading foot. To avoid strain, try to keep your feet within 2.5 cm (1 in) of the ground and your knees slightly bent to absorb impact. Keep your head upright, in line with your spine.

JUMPS
As your fitness level increases begin adding jumps with both feet together. To avoid boredom, you could try some variations such as hopping on one foot, then the other. Again, make sure you do not jump too high. If you keep your feet in fairly close contact with the ground you will minimise the chance of strain and also will be more likely to keep jumping for longer.

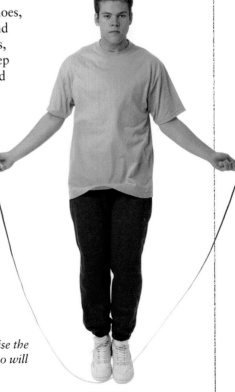

THE STEP TEST

This simple test enables you to assess your aerobic endurance and give you an idea of how fit you really are and what level your exercise programme should take. It is also a useful guide to how your fitness is progressing once your exercise routine has been established.

If your resting heart rate is in the poor range (see page 79) do not attempt the test and seek advice from your doctor. Before you start the test, carry out a 10 minute stretching session to avoid straining yourself. Find a secure step not more than 20–25 cm (8–10 inches) high, stand approximately 30 cm (12 inches) away from it and carry out the test (see right). Check the results against the recovery rate chart on page 79. If you fall in the poor to fair range, you should start an exercise programme very gently.

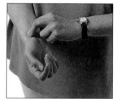

1 *Keep your back straight and stomach in. Step up and down (leading with the right foot up, then the left up, then right down and so on) as fast as is comfortable for three minutes.*

2 *Rest for 30 seconds, and then take your pulse.*

CHARTING PROGRESS
Keeping a record of your exercise regime will help you to measure your progress. Include details of when you exercised, what kind of exercise you performed and for how long, your pulse before and after and your weight. Over a period of a few months of regular exercise you will see an improvement in your resting and recovery heart rates. Avoid weighing yourself too often as daily fluctuations can be misleading.

normal body weight for your height this may also lead to amenorrhea. Consult your doctor if you miss three or more periods.

SETTING UP YOUR OWN EXERCISE PROGRAMME

The first step in setting up your own exercise programme is to find out how fit you are now. Your resting pulse rate already provides some indication of this; but you can also test your endurance by performing the step test (see above). Once your general fitness level is established, you can begin introducing regular exercise at the right level. If you are not very fit, it is important to begin slowly, gradually building up the intensity of the exercise.

While general aerobic exercise will burn calories, you should also consider exercises to improve the muscle tone of specific areas of the body. For example, if you feel your stomach is too flabby, in addition to general aerobic exercise such as walking, consider doing abdominal exercises regularly to strengthen the stomach muscles; this will tighten and flatten your stomach.

Remember that in order to lose weight, you should eat the right amount of calories (see charts, page 49) which are delivered in a low-fat, complex carbohydrate diet.

Exercising for body shape

People who usually follow diet-only weight loss programmes will notice that when they add an exercise programme, their muscles will strengthen and tone at the same time as their bodies are shedding fat. This produces a much healthier-looking end result, particularly for older women who can find they look gaunt and unwell after losing a lot of weight on a diet-only regime.

Because exercise strengthens and tones muscles, it can also be used successfully as a way to give a more defined body shape to people who want to actually gain weight. Concentrating on strength exercises such as lifting weights, is probably the best form of exercise for toning and adding bulk to all the major muscle groups.

DATE	TYPE OF EXERCISE	SESSION DETAILS	RESTING HEART RATE	RECOVERY HEART RATE	STEP TEST RESULTS	WEIGHT (kg)
2 Feb	Skipping	10 mins	84	106	100	63.5
2 Feb	Brisk walk	30 mins	–	–	–	–
3 Feb	Swimming	40 mins	84	104	–	–
3 Feb	Exercises	10 mins	–	–	–	–
5 Feb	Cycle ride	40 mins	83	108	–	–
5 Feb	Exercises	10 mins	–	–	–	–
2 Mar	Jogging	25 mins	79	100	96	61.5

MAKING EXERCISE A HABIT FOR ALL AGES

Once you have reached your target weight, try to maintain exercise as an important part of your daily life. If your lifestyle changes, adapt your exercise plan accordingly.

Keeping to an exercise programme can be difficult so it is important to get support. Getting and keeping fit is essential at any age so try to interest friends and family in sharing your goal.

MOTIVATING AND ENCOURAGING CHILDREN TO EXERCISE

Studies have shown an alarming increase in obesity in children. While children should eat healthily and should not be allowed too many high-fat snacks such as crisps and chocolate, an actual calorie restricted diet can be dangerous because they are still growing. Encouraging children to exercise is the best way to prevent excessive weight gain and to keep them healthy.

You can begin by setting a good example yourself. It is hard to persuade your child to play outside instead of watching television, if you spend most of your own leisure time in front of the television. Investing in bikes and going on regular family cycle rides can be a great exercise plan. Taking your children with you on walks to the shops and walking with them to school rather than using the car are also good ways to establish positive habits at an early age.

Encourage children in any aptitude they may show for a particular sport and work around problems that may stop them from taking part. For example, an asthmatic child may have difficulty breathing while exercising. Increased fitness can improve asthma and the condition should not stop a child enjoying exercise; consult your doctor about asthma management. Swimming has been shown to be less likely than other sports to cause exercise-induced asthma, and as most children love playing in water, it's a great way to introduce exercise. Increasing your child's fitness outside of school will also help them feel more confident about joining in school sport and activities.

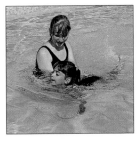

A CONFIDENCE BOOST
Swimming is an excellent exercise for all ages. By introducing them to the sport at an early age you ensure your children do not develop a fear of the water. Once they are competent swimmers, you can take them to a pool with a water slide or a wave machine to keep them amused while you swim some lengths.

EXERCISE AND ASTHMA

In some children and adults, exercise can bring on the wheezing and breathlessness of an asthma attack. This is because exercise increases the flow of air through small airways in the lungs (called bronchioles) causing irritation and narrowing of the airway lining, which restricts the flow of oxygen. Exercising in warm, humid environments reduces the irritation, which makes swimming a good form of exercise for asthmatics. Using a bronchodilator just before exercising also helps to reduce the risk of an asthma attack. Exercise should be avoided in cold or dry conditions.

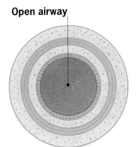

Open airway

HEALTHY BRONCHIOLE
A cross-section through a normal bronchiole shows the rings of muscle and connective tissue in a relaxed, unconstricted state.

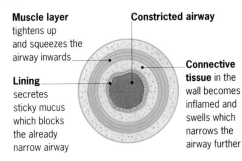

Muscle layer tightens up and squeezes the airway inwards

Lining secretes sticky mucus which blocks the already narrow airway

Constricted airway

Connective tissue in the wall becomes inflamed and swells which narrows the airway further

ASTHMATIC BRONCHIOLE
In an asthma attack, a bronchodilator is used to relax and open the airway. Seek medical attention if it fails to have an effect.

Making exercise fun is the best way to encourage it. If children feel intimidated by the pressure of team sport, explore other exercise options with them. For example, orienteering, where children learn map-reading skills while hiking, may suit a more introverted child. Or try exploiting your child's love of music by taking them to jazz ballet or aerobic classes, or letting them wear a personal stereo while joining in the family walk if this helps to motivate them.

Encourage children to participate in exercises that are appropriate for their age. During early childhood the focus should be on fun games and activities that develop the basic movement skills of running, balancing, jumping, kicking and throwing. Between the ages of 6 and 12 more emphasis can be given to areas where a child shows a particular talent.

Most experts agree that the same level of exercise intensity and frequency used for average adults should be applied to children; that is, low to moderate intensity exercise undertaken for 30 minutes three to four times a week. Children respond to exercise in similar ways to adults and children generally recover from exercise more quickly than adults. But, because children cannot hold as much oxygen in their lungs as adults, they will not be able to match an adult's ability to carry out a prolonged period of exercise. Exercising during very hot weather can also be a problem. As they have lower sweat rates their bodies are less able to cool themselves through evaporation. It is therefore important that children avoid exercise in the middle of the day and to ensure that they drink lots of fluids.

EXERCISING AS YOU GET OLDER
Maintaining an exercise plan as you age has important benefits. Exercising can prevent middle-age spread, slow down stiffening of joints, and relieve other age-related illnesses such as osteoporosis.

DID YOU KNOW?
In 1987, at the age of 67 years and 241 days, Australian swimmer Bertram Clifford Batt became the oldest person ever to swim the English Channel: a distance of some 21 miles (34 km). The swim was completed in a time of 18 hours, 37 minutes.

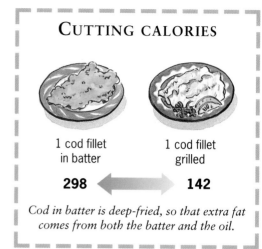

CUTTING CALORIES

1 cod fillet in batter — **298**

1 cod fillet grilled — **142**

Cod in batter is deep-fried, so that extra fat comes from both the batter and the oil.

There is no age limit on exercise and clinical evidence suggests that there need not be a severe decline in fitness with age. In an experiment conducted in a nursing home in 1995 by a specialist in Massachusetts, ten men aged 86 to 96, all of whom had orthopaedic difficulties, volunteered to take up weight training. There were significant gains made in leg muscle strength and size. In 1988, Dr William Evans in the United States, discovered that men aged between 60 and 72 were able to increase their muscular strength by 200 per cent with regular exercise and weight training.

It is wise to consult your doctor before beginning an exercise programme. Avoid very strenuous activities and concentrate on relaxing, gentle forms of exercise. Low-impact exercise (such as swimming or walking) is the most suitable as this places the least stress on joints, and low intensity exercise, which has a lower risk of injury and cardiorespiratory stress, is more appropriate. Tailor exercise to any medical conditions. For example, for people suffering degenerative joint disease, non-weight-bearing activities such as stationary cycling or water exercises are most suitable. Anyone suffering high blood pressure, heart disease or arthritis should avoid weight-lifting exercises as these can place excessive strain on the body.

As the body's thermal control system is less efficient in old age you should avoid exerting the body during extreme weather conditions, opting to exercise in winter during the warmest part of the day, and vice versa in summer. For the same reason dehydration can also be a problem, and drinking plenty of fluids is essential.

CHAPTER 6

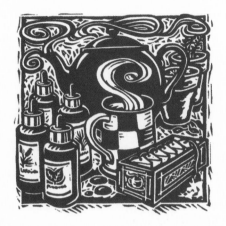

NATURAL THERAPIES AND YOUR WEIGHT

The self-regulating processes of a healthy body will usually keep your weight in the right range, but these can sometimes go wrong for a variety of reasons. Natural therapies work gently on body chemistry, physiology and emotional harmony and, together with an improved diet and an increase in your physical activity, can be used to help restore and maintain a healthy weight.

MIND AND BODY

Natural therapies can help you achieve the goal of successful weight control by combining your physical and mental resources to stimulate the body's in-built self-regulating abilities.

Natural therapies are those that use the resources of nature to promote normal healthy bodily functions. There are many different therapies but all are aimed primarily at encouraging the body's natural mechanisms of self-repair.

Some, such as acupuncture and acupressure, have their origins in antiquity but are applied with more precision in the light of modern knowledge. Others, such as homeopathy and psychotherapy, were developed in recent times by pioneering physicians. Which ones are most appropriate for you will depend on the underlying cause of your body's imbalance.

USING NATURAL THERAPIES

Techniques such as meditation focus on mental and emotional well-being, while others, such as naturopathy, are aimed more at physiological functions, modulating body chemistry by correcting nutritional imbalances or stimulating responses by physical means. For example, a naturopath might recommend changes to your diet as well as suggesting supplements or herbs to assist the metabolism.

Herbal medicine might be helpful where specific organs, such as the liver, are malfunctioning and interfering with the efficient working of the digestive system. Homeopathy, on the other hand, works on both physical and mental levels, with remedies chosen according to the individual's particular temperament and symptoms.

Therapies such as acupuncture and reflexology make use of the network of nerve and energy pathways within the body to regulate mental and physical imbalances.

No short cuts

Many natural therapies can make a positive contribution to weight control but no single system has all the answers. Some are more effective in combination; for example, when herbal medicines are used to reinforce the dietary measures recommended by a naturopath. By including the positive suggestion of hypnotherapy or the insights of counselling you can adopt a much broader approach. These therapies help you to deal with problems such as food cravings, depression and anxiety which may be stopping you from reaching your weight goals.

Natural therapies help you to get the most from your weight-control regime because they are tailored to your individual needs. Whichever you choose, it is essential to combine a well-planned diet with a suitable exercise programme.

ENERGY CENTRES

Developed in ancient India, ayurvedic medicine focuses on seven energy centres (chakras) between the crown and the base of the spine which are believed to be essential to health. Each chakra is linked to one or more parts of the body:

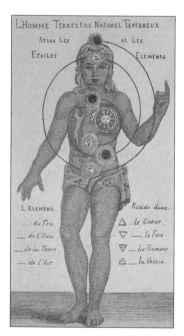

▶ *Sahasrara (crown): whole being.*

▶ *Ajna (brow): brain.*

▶ *Vishuddi (throat): lungs, throat.*

▶ *Anahata (heart): arms, heart.*

▶ *Manipura (solar plexus): small intestine, liver, stomach, spleen.*

▶ *Svadisthana (sacral): reproductive organs, kidneys, bladder.*

▶ *Muladhara (base): large intestine.*

EAST MEETS WEST

This illustration showing the seven chakras comes from the Theosophica Practica, *published by the Theosophical Society which was formed in France in 1875 by Helena Blavatsky to introduce Eastern philosophy to the West.*

Reflexology

Reflexology is an ancient healing art which therapists believe can restore health to organs of the body. It can play an important part in a weight-control programme by improving body functions such as digestion and metabolism.

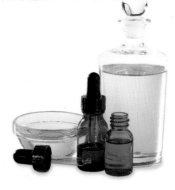

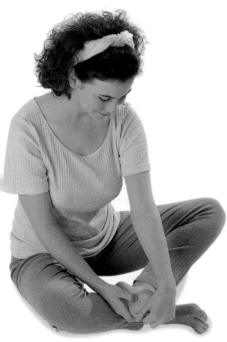

Reflexology is based on the belief that every organ in the body corresponds to zones on the sides and soles of the feet, and that massaging them will promote health.

Sit comfortably on a chair or bed with the feet bare and bend one knee so that you can grasp the foot with both hands.

Using the index or middle fingers, knead the zones shown below; spend up to a minute on each zone. If the area is tender, work gently until it eases. Work on all the relevant zones for a few minutes every day or, if you prefer, select two or three of the zones you feel are the most important for daily attention, treating others once or twice a week as added tonics.

ADDED BENEFIT
Using essential oils as you massage will accentuate the benefits to the organs.

USING ESSENTIAL OILS

Aromatherapy uses essential oils extracted from flowers, plants, trees and spices for their antiseptic and anti-bacterial properties and the therapeutic effects of their scents. Never use oils straight from the bottle and as feet are sensitive, dilute them more than for body massage. Use about one drop of the oil to every 10 ml of base oil such as sweet almond, jojoba, peach kernel oil or wheatgerm.

THUMB WALKING

The most fundamental technique in reflexology, thumb walking, will take practice to perfect. Your thumb may be sore at first until it has increased in strength.

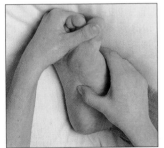

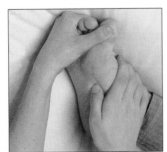

1 *Press the ball of your thumb into the sole of your foot. To move, walk your thumb forward by slightly bending and unbending it at its joint.*

2 *As you walk your thumb towards your toes keep it in gentle contact with the skin. Don't straighten the thumb completely or it will cover areas too quickly.*

ZONES TO TREAT

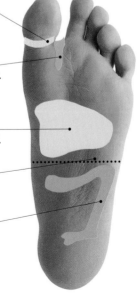

Thyroid – on the soles in a narrow band around the 'neck' of the big toes. Use essential oil of sage here as it is a good general metabolism stimulant

Lymphatic system – between the first and second toes on the tops and soles of the feet. Rub in juniper or lemon oil – both are known for their detoxifying properties

Stomach – the inner square inch on the sole of the left foot between the ball and 'waistline'. Use fennel, cardamom or peppermint oil to ease indigestion and upset stomachs

Waistline

Large intestine – on the soles of the feet in a line of 2.5–5 cm (1–2 in) up the outer side of each foot and across below the 'waistline'. Rose, rosemary and marjoram are good essential oils for this area, easing bowel movement

Therapies for Your Body

Natural therapies that use herbs, flowers, foods and water can play a part in helping you reach your weight goals, especially when used in conjunction with a diet and exercise plan.

Herbal drinks

Health food stores sell some dried medicinal plants for use in infusions. Pour hot water over half a teaspoonful in a small glass of water and leave to infuse for 10-15 minutes. This can be consumed three or four times a day.

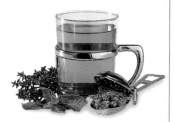

PREPARING AN INFUSION
You can prepare your own herbal drinks at home using fresh herbs – a few leaves of mint, thyme or parsley for example.

Although they are quite diverse in their approaches, natural therapists are united in their belief that health is dependent on the interaction of the body and mind and that it is important to treat the person as a whole and to search out the underlying causes of an illness or condition, rather than just treating the symptoms.

HERBALISM

One of the oldest and most universal forms of medical care is the use of preparations of roots, stems, leaves, flowers and seeds of plants, internally or on the skin. Modern phytotherapy (medical herbalism) uses plants to treat various illnesses and diseases as well as promoting general health and well-being. Herbalists use the whole plant or specific parts, rather than a drug derived from it, because they believe as yet unidentified compounds in the plant may play an important role in the therapeutic effect.

As part of a weight-control programme, herbal medicines can have positive influences on the body's effective functioning, depending on their individual properties. For example, alteratives (which help to remove waste material from various tissues of the body) and diuretics (which increase the elimination of waste fluids) remove the toxic products which might otherwise obstruct normal functioning and lead to the accumulation of weight, especially through fluid retention.

Other herbal treatments assist this detoxification process by promoting the sweating (cleansing) functions of the skin. Apart from this cleansing process, there are other herbal preparations which have properties that act to stimulate body functions which are not working effectively.

Medical herbalists can tailor combinations of herbs to your particular needs. For example, the thyroid gland – which regulates the body's metabolism – is dependent on iodine salts for its effectiveness, and kelp (see box below) can supply these.

As with any medication, it is important not to exceed the recommended dose of herbal medicines and to stop the treatment if there is any sign of an allergic reaction.

THE PROPERTIES OF KELP

Kelp, or bladderwrack, a common species of seaweed, has been used for over 200 years as a tonic for hypothyroidism (see page 34). Its high iodine content stimulates thyroid production, stabilising the metabolism. Kelp can also help hypothyroidism sufferers lose weight by promoting the faster burning of calories. If you have an overactive thyroid, or are allergic to iodine, avoid taking kelp.

A USEFUL SUPPLEMENT
Kelp is available in powder and tablet form from most health food stores. If your thyroid function is normal kelp will not aid weight loss but will still provide useful amounts of iodine, vitamins and minerals.

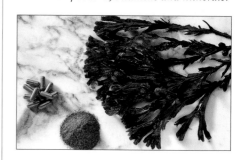

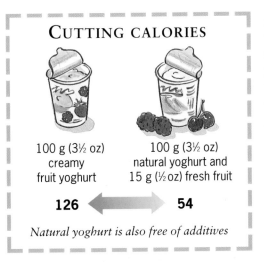

CUTTING CALORIES

100 g (3½ oz)
creamy
fruit yoghurt

100 g (3½ oz)
natural yoghurt and
15 g (½ oz) fresh fruit

126 ⬅➡ **54**

Natural yoghurt is also free of additives

HOMEOPATHY

Homeopathy was founded by the German physician and chemist Samuel Hahnemann in the early 19th century. Today, more than 2000 homeopathic remedies are in use, derived from a range of plant, animal and mineral sources.

While herbal medicines work directly on the physiology of digestion and body function, homeopathic remedies have a more subtle influence on health by stimulating the body's powers of self-healing. The medicinal substance is repeatedly diluted by a special process until there is no trace of the active ingredient remaining that can be detected by normal chemical analysis. Homeopaths believe that the greater the dilution of a remedy the more powerful it becomes and the more carefully it must be matched to the symptoms and the characteristics of the patient. These 'high potency' remedies are, therefore, best prescribed by qualified homeopaths, but many lower potency preparations are widely available in chemists and health food stores as single remedies or combinations for particular health needs.

Selecting the right remedy

At a consultation with a qualified homeopath you will be asked a variety of questions ranging well beyond those which seem relevant to your weight problem. Your response to environmental changes, foods, sleeping habits, temperament, and many other factors can all help the practitioner to select the most appropriate treatment. Having chosen one or more remedies, these may be prescribed in a suitable potency (dilution), usually made up in tablet form.

Homeopathic medicines in low potencies are very safe and may be purchased from homeopathic pharmacies or some chemists. Because the active ingredient in homeopathic medicines has been greatly diluted, it is easily neutralised by strong tasting or strongly aromatic substances such as spicy foods, alcohol, tobacco, tea and coffee and toothpaste. For this reason you will be instructed to take your medicines well apart from mealtimes, drinks, and brushing your teeth.

FLOWER REMEDIES FOR MIND AND MOOD

Bach flower remedies combine the theories of homeopathy and herbal medicine. They are named after their originator, Dr Edward Bach, who believed that certain flowers found in the European countryside can help to reduce emotional states such as impatience, fear, timidity, grief or lack of motivation. As research has shown a link between an individual's emotional state and food cravings, Bach flower remedies may assist in tackling the emotional issues that are often the root cause of overeating.

Bach flower remedies are prepared by distilling freshly picked flower heads in bowls of spring water that are left in direct sunlight. They are sold in many pharmacies and health food stores.

Some of the following remedies may be of benefit to people with weight problems:

▶ *Hornbeam – relieves weariness/mental fatigue.*

▶ *Centaury – increases willpower.*

▶ *Chestnut bud – helps to avoid repetition of mistakes, such as impulsive eating.*

▶ *Wild oat – can be a catalyst for change, helping you to make clear decisions.*

▶ *Pine – may help people who tend to reproach themselves.*

HOW MUCH TO TAKE
To make the standard dosage add 2 drops of the remedy to 30 ml (1 fl oz) water; take 4 drops of this mixture orally four times daily.

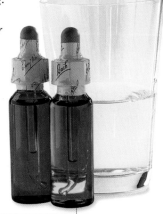

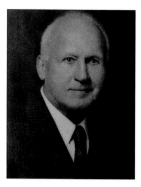

NATURAL PIONEER
German-born Benedict Lust began using the term 'naturopathy' in the USA in 1902. He used the term to describe his vision for the future of natural medicine: a fusing of a diverse range of therapies including herbal medicine, homeopathy, and nutritional therapy.

Homeopathic remedies that may be beneficial as part of a weight-control programme include calcium carbonate, which can assist in reducing water retention, and *Thyroidinum* which can help combat cravings for sweet food.

NATUROPATHY

Naturopathy is a system of medicine which encourages you to take considerable responsibility for your own health. It is based on one basic principle – that all forms of disease are the result of incorrect living habits, particularly with regard to diet. These bad habits result in the accumulation of toxic waste materials which interfere with the body's normal processes.

A qualified naturopath – recognised by the initials ND (Naturopathic Diploma) after their name – will offer you advice about various aspects of health care based on a thorough discussion and medical examination. The treatment recommended will revolve around dietary and nutritional changes, supported by physical measures to stimulate metabolism by encouraging the functions of the skin, lungs, bowels and kidneys which are responsible for removing waste from the body.

There are many types of diet regimes that a naturopath might recommend, depending on your constitution, age and health history. These may include fasting and cleansing diets, which, along with most other strategies that are employed, can be carried out at home as long as you carefully follow the guidelines provided by the naturopath. Some diets may need to be combined with hydrotherapy techniques. A naturopath might also prescribe enzyme preparations, herbs, or supplements to assist the digestion and improve the metabolism.

The use of hydrotherapy

Many naturopaths employ hydrotherapy, the healing techniques using water, as part of their treatment programmes. Various forms of hydrotherapy are recommended to help the skin to function more efficiently. Some treatments such as hot and cold compresses, friction rubs and seaweed baths can be done at home (see right).

The skin is an important organ with the ability to absorb substances (for example, through aromatherapy) in addition to its vital function of eliminating toxic waste products through perspiration. It is also connected by nerve pathways to internal organs such as the liver and kidneys. Therefore stimulation of the skin can have many positive benefits in your overall health. A body that is functioning more efficiently will also enhance your weight-control programme.

Residential care

There are a few centres in the UK and the rest of Europe, Australia, and USA where residential treatment can be given under naturopathic medical supervision. These clinics provide dietary treatment, massage, reflex therapies, and hydrotherapy, using more sophisticated equipment for baths, sprays, and steam cabinets than would normally be available in the home.

They are often situated in pleasant surroundings where patients can stay for a week or more to detoxify and shed surplus weight, while learning how to continue to follow a new, healthier lifestyle once they have returned home.

Pathway to health

Hydrotherapy techniques that can be of help to people with weight problems include hot and cold compresses, friction rubs and seaweed baths.

Hot and cold compresses are easy to apply at home and can be used to stimulate blood flow to internal organs such as the liver and stomach – apply a damp towel, soaked in hot water, to the upper abdominal area for about 3 minutes, then one soaked in cold water for 1 minute.

A friction rub stimulates the blood circulation, boosts the immune system, and helps the skin shed dead cells. After a hot bath or shower, soak a loofah in cold water and give the body a firm rub down.

A seaweed bath – soaking for 20-30 minutes in a hot bath to which seaweed extract has been added – induces increased perspiration and the uptake of natural iodine, and other mineral compounds, which helps stimulate the thyroid gland. Avoid if you have hyperthyroidism.

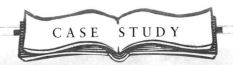

The Overeater

The urge to overeat may arise for a number of reasons, both physical and emotional. Metabolic imbalances can create a vicious circle of craving inappropriate foods or abnormal hunger that may, in turn, affect physical and mental energy. An approach that includes improvements in diet and addresses the underlying psychological factors is essential.

Walter, a 43-year-old marketing manager, was recently warned about his weight during a routine check-up for an insurance policy. His weight and blood pressure have been steadily creeping up and he now realises that as he ages, he can no longer indulge in business meals and between-meal snacks as he has in the past. Previously, whenever he has tried any form of slimming diet, he has become tired and irritable, his hunger has increased and inevitably he reverted to eating unsuitable foods and regained any weight he had lost. Walter is concerned that his rising weight is beginning to affect his health. His GP has suggested that a naturopath might be able to help.

WHAT SHOULD WALTER DO?

After a thorough examination and blood and sweat tests, which revealed shortages of minerals and trace elements that help control the level of fat and cholesterol, the naturopath gave Walter specific advice about his diet.

Walter needs to eat well-balanced meals that sustain his metabolism for longer periods and remove the need for unhealthy snacks while also reducing his calorie intake. Complex carbohydrates, vegetables, salads and fresh fruit should replace fatty and sugary snacks.

The naturopath explained to Walter how he might benefit his body with his mind (see page 96) and suggested the use of simple hydrotherapy at home (see page 92).

Action Plan

DIET
Replace fats and sugary snacks with fruits and vegetables. Include more complex carbohydrates in meals for sustained energy.

EMOTIONAL HEALTH
Use visualisation and meditation to focus on weight-loss goals and improve motivation.

HEALTH
After a morning shower or bath, use a loofah loaded with cold water to briskly rub the skin. This stimulates blood circulation and the effectiveness of the kidneys, liver and lungs.

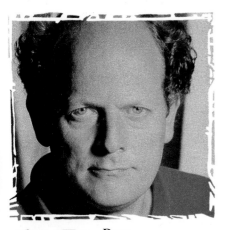

DIET
Insufficient energy from the right kind of food can lead to frequent snacking and overeating.

EMOTIONAL HEALTH
A negative attitude to dieting can lead to failure in weight-control plans. Walter has to believe that his weight goals are achievable to increase his motivation.

HEALTH
Inefficient elimination of waste products and fluid can cause an imbalance in metabolism. Natural therapies such as hydrotherapy may help to overcome this.

HOW THINGS TURNED OUT FOR WALTER

By eating regular meals based on healthy eating principles, Walter began to feel more energetic and lost his tendency to snack during the day. The naturopath prescribed a chromium supplement to help lower his blood pressure and aid glucose metabolism. His cold friction rub in the morning braced him for the day ahead. As he lost weight and felt healthier, his concentration at work improved and he even began an exercise programme.

THERAPIES FOR ENERGY BALANCING

Eastern therapies such as acupuncture are based on the belief that any health problem can be improved by balancing the flow of energy through the body's network of energy pathways.

Many therapies aim to restore good health by treating imbalances in the nerve and energy paths within the body. Reflexology, for example, can be used to aid relaxation and help you to prepare your state of mind before beginning a weight-control programme.

ACUPUNCTURE

Acupuncture is a form of therapy in which fine needles are applied to acupoints on the body. This network of points lies along a series of channels, or meridians, situated just beneath the skin which, in turn, are connected by internal pathways to the major organs. The whole network, which is distinct from the nerves, blood vessels, and lymph channels, makes up an energy system that is believed to regulate all bodily functions. Acupoints are identified by their meridian names (usually that of an associated organ) and a number.

There is some scientific evidence to support acupuncture. It is known that applying needles to acupoints on the skin causes the body to release 'feel-good' hormones (called endorphins). However, while this might account for some of the benefits achieved by acupuncture, it cannot explain other metabolic changes that a qualified practitioner may be able to initiate.

Acupuncture may help to tackle weight problems by improving general well-being, overcoming fatigue, harmonising digestive functions, reducing tension and anxiety, regulating fluid balance and controlling the tendency for food cravings.

ACUPRESSURE

It is probable that acupuncture developed out of an older system known as acupressure or shiatsu. Acupressure also involves acupoints but, as the name suggests, uses pressure rather than needles. It is believed that regular massage of acupoints may act as a tonic to the organs or functions with which they are connected.

Acupressure is best carried out with the tip of the thumb or middle finger or with a rounded device such as a pen top. To stimulate a particular organ or part of the body, apply slow steady pressure and gentle circular kneading movements to the relevant acupoint for one to two minutes at a time. A calming and sedating effect is achieved by applying firm, deep, pressure, sustained for a longer period – two or three minutes.

TREATING CRAVINGS WITH EAR THERAPY

Auricular, or ear, acupuncture is a specialised therapy based on the principle that points on the outer ear relate to each of the major organs. The pattern formed by these points is believed to mirror the position of a foetus in the womb.

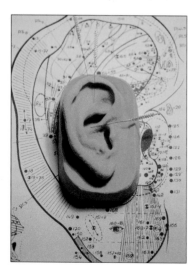

EAR ACUPUNCTURE
Auricular acupuncture uses 120 points on the ear to regulate all other parts of the body. Tiny 'press needles' are inserted by the practitioner and retained under a waterproof plaster for up to two weeks. The patient is instructed to press on the needles several times a day – pressure is barely felt. Practitioners believe that stimulation of the points connected with the digestive organs can help to control addictive tendencies such as food cravings.

ACUPRESSURE FOR WEIGHT CONTROL

Acupressure may help weight control by freeing blocked energy channels and so restoring the healthy functioning of the digestive organs. To stimulate one of the pressure points below, simply apply slow, steady pressure from the thumb or middle finger. Maintain pressure for 20 seconds and release for 10 – repeat this process up to a maximum time of 3 minutes on each point and practise daily.

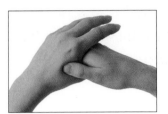

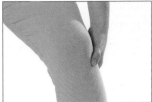

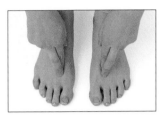

PRESSURE POINT LI 4
To improve bowel function, apply pressure to the back of the hand in the soft flesh between the thumb and index finger.

PRESSURE POINT ST 36
To stimulate digestion and metabolism, apply pressure four finger widths below the knee, towards the outside of the shin bone.

PRESSURE POINT LIV 3
To stimulate the function of the liver, apply pressure to the foot in the angle between the first and second metatarsal bones.

Before selecting the appropriate points, a practitioner of acupuncture or acupressure will make a careful assessment of a patient's needs using the principles of traditional Chinese medicine (TCM). This determines the balance of energy flow or evidence of sluggishness in particular parts of the body.

A blockage in the abdominal area, for example, can prevent proper digestive function, causing excess energy to flow upwards and leading to heat or flushing in the head or face. In this case, the practitioner will select acupoints principally on the arms, legs, and abdomen.

At the other extreme, energy depletion can lead to fluid retention. In this case the practitioner may apply heat to the acupoints by burning a herb called moxa. This technique, called moxibustion, is an invaluable part of TCM which may assist the overweight individual. The treatment increases the general energy and efficiency of the digestive organs and improves metabolism thereby benefiting any patient who is undergoing a diet and exercise programme.

REFLEXOLOGY

There are many areas on the surface of the body that have special points (called reflex points or zones) that correspond to internal organs. One of the most accessible areas with reflex zones is the soles of the feet. In the 1930s, Eunice Ingham, a New York therapist, rediscovered a system of connecting reflex foot zones to the rest of the body which she called reflexology. This system had also been known to the ancient Chinese and Egyptians. Ingham found that by massaging the tender areas of the feet she could influence the organs connected with them.

The foot zones occupy large areas of the soles, particularly where larger organs like the liver are concerned, so they are relatively easy to locate and manipulate (see page 89).

BURNING OFF CALORIES: *Squash*

A very intense game, squash sharpens the reflexes and demands high energy expenditure and concentration. A good cardiovascular exercise, it will improve endurance, agility and strength.

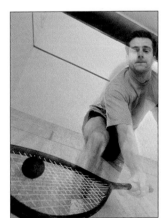

MUSCLE GROUPS BENEFITING
Legs, lower torso and arm muscles are all utilised during a game.

EQUIPMENT
A court and partner is required, with racquets and squash balls. Light, comfortable clothing is most suitable.

CALORIES BURNT
Playing squash burns about ten calories a minute (600 an hour).

THERAPIES FOR YOUR MIND

Mood and motivation are such important aspects of weight regulation that mental factors must always be considered alongside diet and fitness improvements.

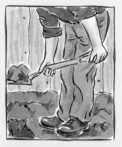

QUICK FITNESS TIP
Take an active interest in your garden. As well as burning energy, gardening can also help to lift your mood.

Whether you need to strengthen your resolve or deal with the deeper emotional conflicts which underlie eating disorders, there are numerous therapies that work with the mind and may assist resolution of weight problems.

MEDITATION

The term 'meditation' covers a wide range of practices from simple prayer to the esoteric exercises of transcendental meditation. The principle aim of meditation is to bring the mind under control and to focus it in order to free it of negative thoughts and emotions. Meditation is a therapeutically broad approach which may be used in many techniques including autogenics, hypnotherapy,

behavioural psychology and psychotherapy. Most forms of meditation are carried out in a relatively passive state. Some, however, involve gentle movement or even quite vigorous physical exercise – 'dynamic meditation' – such as that used by the 'Whirling Dervishes', a Muslim sect who achieve a trance state through spinning dances. A meditative element also forms an integral part of oriental practices, such as yoga, t'ai chi and qigong, where breathing and rhythmical movement are used to harmonise body and mind.

Other Eastern-based systems of meditation use a mantra – a chant or rhyme on which the individual should focus when meditating. Concentrating on a mantra helps to block out intrusive thoughts and calms the mind. A similar principle is used in the meditative technique of visualisation.

Visualisation

Mental imagery, or creative visualisation, can be a healthy way of ridding the body of negative images and stress and can be harnessed to produce a positive frame of mind. In a study carried out in the 1970s, US cancer specialist, Dr Carl Simonton, found that patients undergoing conventional cancer treatment had a better survival rate when they spent some time each day focusing on their bodies' healing processes at work using mental images to which they could relate. For some, a military analogy might work, by imagining the white blood cells as an army advancing on the tumour and overwhelming it. A young child may picture a team of dwarfs shovelling away the growth.

This technique can be applied to many aspects of health, including weight problems. It doesn't have to be a biologically

HOW TO MEDITATE

Meditation is easy to do at home and anything up to one hour of meditation each day can be beneficial during a weight-control plan by boosting positivity. Sitting comfortably with your back straight, breathe steadily and focus your mind on your breath as it flows in and out of your lungs. After a few minutes, visualise pleasant, tranquil surroundings, such as the sea shore or a woodland riverside. Playing tapes of soothing music may also help to create the right mood.

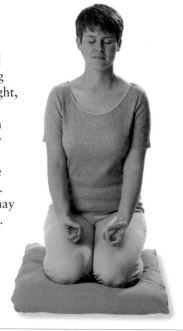

FINDING A POSITION
Adopt a comfortable position which allows you to breathe freely and deeply.

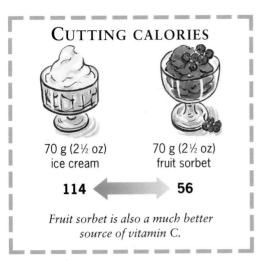
correct image. Just the process of regular visualisation can initiate positive changes. For example, the overweight individual can visualise fatty tissues dissolving away and being carried out of the body. Or they may use visualisation to 'create' a goal for weight loss by visualising themselves exactly as they would like to be. They could also use visualisation to discourage unhealthy eating by imagining what that chocolate bar or packet of crisps will do to their body. Visualisation is only limited by imagination.

HYPNOTHERAPY

The power of the mind can be harnessed for healing and self-development in a number of ways but hypnotherapy can achieve this in a more positive way for individuals who may find meditation and visualisation difficult to sustain. In hypnotherapy an altered state of consciousness is induced by the practitioner who then offers positive suggestions to the patient. For people with weight problems these may centre on understanding and overcoming addictive tendencies. Hypnotherapy became popular with many psychologists in the 1800s (but lost favour at the turn of the century) as a means of getting faster results and more accurate analysis of the patient's problems. While in the trance-like state induced by the hypnotherapist the patient is open to suggestions from the practitioner and to the free expression of his or her own emotions.

When the therapist wishes to impart positive suggestions to a patient who needs to exercise dietary restraint, the removal of some mental resistance to these ideas can be a great advantage. It can also clear the way for a more relaxed discussion of emotional conflicts, which may underlie cravings, bingeing habits, or other eating disorders.

Contrary to popular belief hypnotherapy does not generally entail a loss of control over your own mind, merely a release of some of your emotional inhibitions.

Autosuggestion

The principle of reinforcing the motivation of the mind by repeating positive suggestion to yourself was first developed by Emile Coué. He encouraged patients to set aside times for mental concentration when they could repeat phrases which were appropriate to their needs. His most famous term – a type of mantra – was: 'Every day, in every way, I am getting better and better'. Coué's objective was to stimulate the patient's

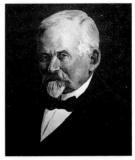

*EMILE COUÉ
A French apothecary, Coué (1857-1926) became interested in autosuggestion when a patient's chronic illness was cured by a 'new medicine' which turned out to be just coloured water. Now known as the placebo effect, this showed Coué how the mind has the ability to influence the physical condition of the body.*

THE STATE OF HYPNOTIC TRANCE

The state of trance induced during a hypnotherapy session is similar to daydreaming or sleepwalking. Therapists use this state to confront underlying emotional problems that may be causing physical symptoms in the patient.

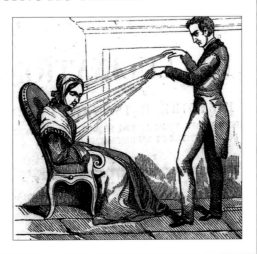

*MESMERISM AND MODERN HYPNOTHERAPY
This picture, dating from about 1840, shows the 'lines of force' that were believed to 'mesmerise' the patient into a state of trance. Today, hypnosis is thought to work by inducing an altered state of highly relaxed consciousness where the deepest recesses of the mind are made accessible.*

GOALS FOR CHANGE

Cognitive behaviour therapy may help to motivate you towards your weight goals by prompting some positive changes.

▶ *A way of acting – to be more outgoing and confident about your self-image.*

▶ *A way of feeling – to be more positive.*

▶ *A way of thinking – to recognise and solve the underlying causes of your weight problem by employing positive thinking instead of negative.*

▶ *A way of coping – to take charge of your health, and work towards improving your eating habits.*

imagination and concentrate his or her mind. The principle could equally well be applied to the needs of a person with weight problems: 'Every day, in every way, I am getting slimmer and trimmer'.

Autogenic training is a modern variation of this. It uses techniques that must be taught by an expert which enable the individual to focus the mind in order to influence the body. These techniques include a series of basic exercises, such as imagining the arms growing heavy, coupled with a process of mental visualisation of wellness.

BEHAVIOURAL THERAPY

The capacity of the mind to learn new skills is the principle behind behavioural therapy, a form of psychology based on a theory of learning. There are certain patterns of behaviour which can underlie various types of eating disorders, such as anorexia, bulimia, and bingeing habits. Just as you learn the essentials of social conduct throughout childhood by observing adults around you and receiving positive or negative reinforcements from them, so you can also be taught to change patterns of behaviour that develop in adolescence or adulthood.

Certain situations give rise to nervous responses such as panic, fear, guilt and depression. These reactions can be modified, thus enabling the patient to adapt to new stimuli or eradicate old problem traits of behaviour. The origins of behavioural psychology lie in the experiments carried out by the Russian physiologist Ivan Pavlov (see

box, below) who trained dogs to associate the sound of a bell with the imminent arrival of their food until they eventually salivated in response to the bell alone, even when no food was forthcoming.

Cognitive behavioural therapy is one of the related forms of psychotherapy that is practised today and which focuses mainly on the patient's present attitude rather than reaching back into his or her past. The aim of this form of therapy is to teach the patient how to break out of the negative thought patterns that may be underlying destructive forms of behaviour such as bingeing, and to begin to view themselves in a more positive light (see left).

Overcoming weight-related anxieties

Whether you are underweight or overweight, eating too little or too much, or bingeing and vomiting (bulimia), there could be significant emotional factors responsible for your actions, so you may find it necessary to get professional guidance.

Behavioural psychotherapy can help with all types of eating disorders. For example, it can help obese patients by education and reinforcement of healthy eating habits. For anorexic patients, the therapist concentrates on the root of the disease – the patient's negative self-image. By cultivating a habit to consume a healthy diet and avoid bingeing, therapy may help those suffering from bulimia by reducing and eventually preventing the 'guilt' responses which cause the individual to vomit away the calories.

Origins

Russian scientist Ivan Petrovich Pavlov discovered the conditioned reflex, showing the connection between external stimuli and physiological responses. His lifetime's study was concentrated on the blood pressure, digestion and nervous system of dogs. His ground-breaking research into the learned response of dogs showed how animals (and by implication, humans) can learn patterns of behaviour that quickly become powerful and hard-to-change habits (such as bingeing, a characteristic of bulimia nervosa). His influence is still present in modern-day behavioural psychology.

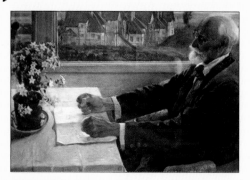

IVAN PAVLOV
Pavlov (1849-1936) pioneered research into learned bodily responses, for which he received a Nobel prize in 1904.

CHAPTER 7

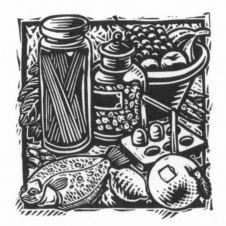

THE PROS AND CONS OF DIETS

The pressure to conform to the ideal slim physique, together with concerns over the negative health consequences of obesity, has led to an array of slimming techniques, books, programmes and aids that all promise rapid and successful weight loss. Many studies have reported that dieting is on the increase, with more than half the adults in the UK trying to diet each year. In spite of this obesity is rising rapidly.

FACTS AND FALLACIES OF DIETING

Healthy eating habits are essential to avoid developing a pattern of bingeing and dieting that is not only an inefficient way to lose weight but can also lead to physical and emotional side effects.

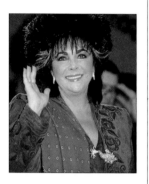

STAR'S STRUGGLE
Elizabeth Taylor's struggle to stay slim in order to conform to an idealised Hollywood film star image has resulted in a pattern of weight gain and dieting that is a classic symptom of weight cycling.

There is a common misconception that overweight people are much more unhealthy than their slim counterparts. While it is true that obesity is harmful, being underweight carries its own health risks (see page 20). Women, for example, need a certain amount of body fat for normal reproductive function, which is why they lay down more fat than men during adolescence.

THE DIET INDUSTRY'S INFLUENCE

The highly lucrative diet industry tends to exploit the public's fears with myths about obesity and dieting that are not always backed up by science. It also encourages the pursuit of unhealthy slenderness. Current expert opinion suggests that some diet plans are not scientifically valid and may be dangerous. In such cases the risk of the diet may outweigh the risks of being moderately overweight. These diets often only work in the short term with weight being quickly regained when normal eating is resumed.

DIETING AND YOUR BODY

Dieting, especially strict dieting, causes you to disregard natural hunger signals from your body. This can have a severe effect on your metabolism and even cause emotional disturbances. For example, many people find that they develop an abnormal preoccupation with food which affects their social behaviour.

There is plenty of evidence that when people go on a diet their body compensates by conserving energy, particularly during fasting or severe calorie restriction. The weight loss that occurs on a crash diet is short-lived because it is mainly water and protein from the muscle that has been shed, rather than excess fat.

It is extremely difficult to maintain a very low level of food intake over a long period of time, and most people find that they quickly return to their normal pattern of eating. In most cases, any weight lost is soon regained.

DIETS AND RELIGION

Many religions impose permanent or temporary dietary rules and recommendations on adherents. Roman Catholics, for example, are asked to give up a favourite food during Lent. Fasting is also important in many faiths as a sign of reverence or self-discipline.

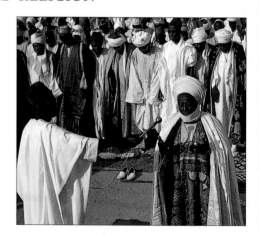

END OF RAMADAN
Moslems fast during Ramadan in the hope of their sins being pardoned. Even water is excluded during daylight hours. This picture shows the traditional prayer ceremony that marks the conclusion of the festival.

CAUTION
If you have a health problem you should consult your doctor before starting a diet of any kind. Pregnant women, children and the elderly should seek guidance from a dietitian instead of dieting.

Risks of weight cycling

Someone who is intent on losing weight can end up in a cycle of recurrent weight gains and losses known as weight cycling, or 'yo-yo dieting'. Weight loss is rarely maintained in the long term and frequent fluctuations in weight are common.

There can be serious health risks from this type of dieting such as irregularities in heart rate that can lead to sudden heart attacks, and a loss of minerals from the bones. Some studies also suggest that people whose weight is constantly fluctuating are at greater risk of heart disease.

The psychological damage of weight cycling may be greater than the physical damage. Repeated cycles of weight loss and regain can contribute to the negative state of mind experienced by chronic dieters, as successful weight loss is followed by a sense of failure when weight is regained as well as feelings of guilt and consequent bingeing.

Chronic dieters are also more likely to feel insecure and have lower self-esteem than non-dieters and are likely to eat more when anxious or depressed than non-dieters. This makes them more vulnerable to social and environmental influences which can lead to extremes in eating behaviour. They are also more susceptible than non-dieters to unrealistic images presented in the media such as models in magazines.

Dieting has been implicated as the starting point for eating disorders such as anorexia nervosa and bulimia nervosa. Both conditions often begin with a simple attempt to lose weight. There are now many self-help organisations providing help for those who find it hard to give up dieting and return to a healthy eating pattern.

A SENSIBLE APPROACH

Drastic measures are not only unlikely to work, but can be dangerous. Crash dieting is not the solution. In fact, long-term weight loss and maintenance can only be achieved by making long-term changes to your lifestyle and eating habits. A nutritionally balanced diet is essential for well-being and must not be compromised for unattainable weight goals. The good news is that current recommendations for healthy eating – a diet low in fat (particularly the saturated type) and high in fibre – can help you to lose weight sensibly. A diet that is high in fat is more likely to cause weight gain than a diet that is high in complex carbohydrates. This is because dietary fat is more likely to be stored by the body, whereas carbohydrates have a limited storage capacity and are rapidly used up for energy production. Switch to lean meat and low-fat products and ensure that the bulk of your diet consists of fruit, vegetables and starchy foods, such as bread, pasta and rice.

This healthy approach to eating not only helps you to lose weight, but may prevent some diseases, such as heart disease and cancer, that can occur in later life. Eating a wide variety of foods will ensure a balanced diet that provides all the nutrients, vitamins and minerals essential for health (see page 51). A diet rich in fruit and vegetables and starchy foods is also thought to protect against intestinal disorders including bowel cancer. An increase in physical activity, which should accompany a healthy eating plan, will reduce the loss of bone mineral – which leads to osteoporosis – and will also help to promote weight loss and well-being.

BURNING OFF CALORIES: *Jogging*

Regular jogging can boost your cardiovascular and respiratory systems, improve your aerobic endurance, and tone and strengthen your muscles. Always introduce a programme gradually.

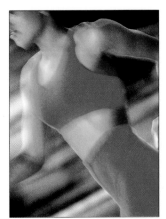

MUSCLE GROUPS BENEFITING
All leg muscles will benefit, but especially the thigh and calf muscles.

EQUIPMENT
Quality running shoes with arch support and cushioned sole are vital to soften the impact. Thick socks help to avoid blisters.

CALORIES BURNT
Jogging for 30 minutes at 11 km (7 miles) per hour will burn 360 Calories (12 Calories per minute).

DIETS FOR MEDICAL REASONS

Many medical conditions can be improved by following special dietary guidelines; for those who have a weight problem as well, it is vital to plan the diet with extra care.

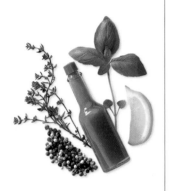

SALT ALTERNATIVES
Excess salt in the diet can aggravate hypertension. Replace it with healthier flavour enhancers, such as peppercorns, lemon, tabasco, or fresh herbs like thyme and basil.

With some disorders, following a strict dietary regime can be a crucial factor in determining whether an individual suffers serious physical symptoms or remains fit and well.

DIABETES MELLITUS

This condition affects one person in 50 in the UK, although many more cases go undiagnosed. Dietary needs vary between sufferers depending on the type of diabetes and whether or not the individual is overweight. However, all diabetics need to follow a diet that is high in complex carbohydrates and low in sugars. This helps to prevent fluctuations in blood glucose levels which cause hypoglycaemia (low blood sugar) or hyper-

glycaemia (high blood sugar). A high fibre intake also slows down the rate of absorption of glucose into the bloodstream and helps to maintain normal blood glucose levels. Limiting fat in the diet to about 30 to 35 per cent of total intake is also recommended to prevent cardiovascular problems that are common in people with diabetes.

HIGH CHOLESTEROL

Individuals with high blood cholesterol, or hypercholesterolaemia, can lower lipid levels by as much as 14 per cent if they adhere to a diet that is low in saturated fats. Meat and full-fat dairy products all contain high levels of saturated fatty acids. People with severe hypercholesterolaemia may also need

SYMPTOMS AND SIGNS OF DIABETES MELLITUS

Diabetes occurs when the pancreas fails to produce enough of the hormone insulin, which the body uses to draw energy from sugar and carbohydrate foods. There are two types of diabetes: the most serious is the insulin-dependent form when a daily injection of insulin is necessary. This type usually develops before the age of 16 and leads to many of the symptoms shown right. Non-insulin-dependent diabetes, which mainly affects the over-40s, can usually be controlled without the need of insulin if a healthy diet is adhered to.

TAKING ACTION
Diabetes is a serious disease and the symptoms shown here call for immediate medical advice. If you experience any of these signs, consult your doctor.

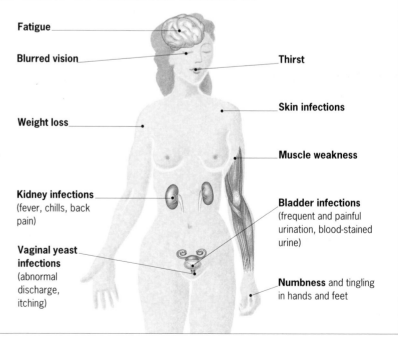

Fatigue

Blurred vision

Thirst

Skin infections

Weight loss

Muscle weakness

Kidney infections
(fever, chills, back pain)

Bladder infections
(frequent and painful urination, blood-stained urine)

Vaginal yeast infections
(abnormal discharge, itching)

Numbness and tingling in hands and feet

CUTTING CHOLESTEROL

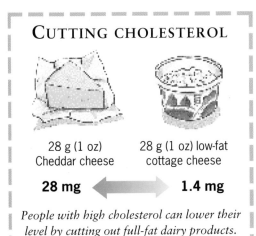

28 g (1 oz)
Cheddar cheese

28 g (1 oz) low-fat
cottage cheese

28 mg ⬅➡ **1.4 mg**

People with high cholesterol can lower their level by cutting out full-fat dairy products.

to take cholesterol-lowering drugs to reduce the risk of cardiovascular disease. Increasing your intake of soluble fibre (found in oats, beans and pulses, fruits and vegetables) can help to lower cholesterol levels by preventing its absorption by the body.

HIGH BLOOD PRESSURE

Cutting down on the saturated fat in your diet is essential in order to lower high blood pressure (hypertension). People at risk of hypertension can also benefit from reducing the salt (sodium) in their diet. Current advice recommends cutting down to 6 g a day from the average daily intake of 9 g. Those taking anti-hypertensive drugs can reduce their blood pressure further by modest reductions in salt intake. Eating plenty of fruit and vegetables also provides potassium, which can counteract some of the negative effects of sodium.

COELIAC DISEASE

Special diets that exclude gluten are essential for people with coeliac disease. This condition is caused by a sensitivity to the protein gluten and affects around one in 1500 people in the UK. In those affected, gluten damages the lining of the small intestine, leading to impaired absorption of nutrients. Symptoms and signs can include diarrhoea, bloating, weight loss and anaemia. Keeping to gluten-free foods can quickly reverse symptoms. Gluten is present in wheat, rye, barley and oats and all foods containing these cereals. Cakes, biscuits, pasta, foods coated with batter or breadcrumbs, soups and breakfast cereals can all contain the protein. Alternative sources of energy and nutrients include pulses, rice,

potatoes, corn (maize) and nuts. Gluten-free bread and other cereals are also available from health food stores. A dietitian can help you to plan a balanced diet that includes all the vital nutrients in the required amounts.

FOOD ALLERGY/INTOLERANCE

People suffering from food intolerance or allergy will improve once they exclude the problem food from their diet. Symptoms of food allergy or intolerance often include excessive tiredness, diarrhoea, migraine and even potentially fatal reactions such as anaphylactic shock. Common culprits include milk, eggs, fish, shellfish, nuts, soya beans and some food additives. Often it is difficult to pinpoint the exact cause and an elimination diet may be necessary. This involves excluding all but a few known 'safe' foods from the diet and then gradually reintroducing other foods to see which ones cause a reaction. This approach requires patience and will-power to succeed. The advice of a doctor or dietitian is also essential to avoid any health risk caused by the restricted diet.

KIDNEY COMPLAINTS

People with kidney problems may need to follow a low-protein diet to prevent further damage to their kidneys. Sodium, potassium and fluids may also have to be restricted in certain patients, depending on the condition and the extent of kidney damage. These diets require professional advice from a dietician as well as plenty of motivation and perseverance from the patient as they are very difficult to follow.

CYSTIC FIBROSIS

People with cystic fibrosis are recommended to follow a high-energy, high-protein diet. This hereditary condition is caused by defective genes inherited from both parents and results in an overproduction of mucus in the lungs and the pancreas. Food is not properly digested and passes into the large bowel, causing diarrhoea and deficiencies in the fat-soluble vitamins A, D, E and K. Apart from taking pancreatic enzymes in capsule form to aid digestion, a diet high in energy, particularly in the form of fat, is essential to meet high nutritional demands. The need to maintain adequate nutrient levels and prevent weight loss far outweighs any increased risk of cardiovascular disease from following a high-fat diet.

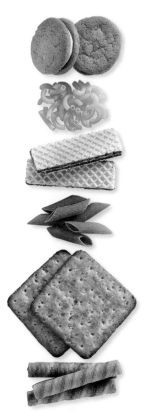

GLUTEN-FREE FOODS
People with coeliac disease, who cannot eat cereal-based products containing gluten, need not miss out on tasty treats. A range of gluten-free sweet biscuits and savoury snacks are available from larger pharmacies and most health food shops.

103

CHOOSING A DIET

To be useful, a diet should promote steady, gradual weight loss and a long-term change to healthy eating habits. It is essential to look beyond the hype and judge a diet's merits for yourself.

Low-fat foods that fill you up

Complex carbohydrates such as potatoes, bread, pasta and cereal should form part of any balanced diet. They are an excellent source of starch, fibre and protein and are filling foods. Essentially, these are low-fat foods – it is the food that you eat with them (the butter and cheese on a baked potato, the creamy sauce on pasta, the whole milk on cereal) which raises the fat content and calorie count. Choose low-fat options such as tuna for potatoes, tomato-based sauces for pasta, and skimmed or semi-skimmed milk for cereal.

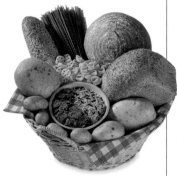

Fibre providers
Fibre is essential to health (see page 49) and can be found in staple foods such as bread, potatoes, rice, cereal and pasta.

Despite the sound dietary guidelines offered by the Health Authority in the UK and the trained dietitians on hand to help individuals with special dietary needs, most people who want to lose weight prefer to follow a published diet. This section of the book examines some of the most popular diets of recent years.

AVOIDING SEVERITY

Some diets have little or no scientific basis and recommend such severe dieting that they can be dangerous to your health. Most can be safely followed for a short amount of time or adapted to avoid health risks.

Fasting

This involves giving up food altogether to achieve rapid weight loss and drinking lots of water during the process. It is sometimes claimed, without scientific proof, that toxins will be flushed out of the body leading to improved health. But totally depriving your body of food for any length of time is dangerous, and in susceptible individuals it can lead to an attack of gout, lowered blood pressure and even heart failure. Often the weight lost is rapidly regained once normal eating resumes. Children, pregnant women and the elderly should never try fasting.

Rotation diet

This diet alternates daily calorie intake from week to week to avoid the metabolic rate decreases believed to occur when a low calorie diet is followed for a long time. Initially 600 calories a day are allowed, followed by 900 and then 1200 – the cycle is repeated until the desired weight is achieved.

There is no scientific evidence that the body's metabolism can be tricked in this way and reducing intake to 600 calories a day makes it difficult to ensure you get all the vitamins and minerals that you need.

Mono-diets

These diets are based on one food, which is allowed in unlimited amounts to the virtual exclusion of everything else. These 'wonder' foods are claimed to contain substances that enhance the fat-burning process and speed weight loss. Fruits such as pineapple and papaya have been cited but while it is true that they contain enzymes that can break up proteins, there is no evidence that they aid the digestive system in any way. There is no 'magic' involved – the restricted food choice makes it very hard to consume a lot of calories so some weight loss is inevitable, particularly if it is a low-calorie food. These diets are generally not recommended as they are far too low in energy and no single food can provide all the nutrients necessary for a balanced diet.

Scarsdale diet

This diet recommends plenty of protein in the form of poultry, fish and eggs. It provides around 43 per cent of calories from protein, while the current recommendation suggests 10 to 15 per cent as being adequate. Fats and carbohydrates are also limited on this diet, but there is no restriction on any lean protein food. It is suggested that the diet should not be followed for longer than 14 days – few people can resolve their weight problem this quickly.

Low carbohydrate diet

This type of diet aims to restrict the intake of carbohydrate-rich foods such as bread, potatoes, pasta and rice. The principle behind it is that once you cut out starchy foods from the diet, the energy intake is automatically reduced. However, the fat intake tends to be high on this diet which goes against the current recommendations for reducing heart disease. Also many people feel hungry between meals.

THE HAY DIET

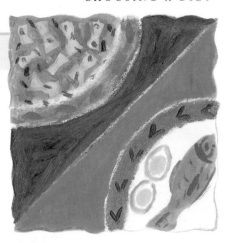

The theory that proteins and carbohydrates should not be mixed in the same meal was made popular by Dr William Hay, in the early 1900s. He believed that conditions such as indigestion, allergies and skin disorders were due to an accumulation of toxins in the body caused by eating too much meat and processed foods. His diet recommends that vegetables, salads and fruits form the bulk of the diet while concentrated sources of proteins, carbohydrates and fats are consumed sparingly. Carbohydrate foods such as potatoes and pasta should not be eaten in the same meal as protein foods such as meat and dairy products. Meals should be at least four hours apart to allow digestion.

Rationale
The theory of this diet is that for digestion carbohydrates need an alkaline environment while proteins require acidic conditions. Mixing the two is said to neutralise the medium causing malabsorption and inadequate digestion. Scientists today discredit this theory – many foods contain both carbohydrates and proteins and the digestive system handles both simultaneously.

Risks
This diet perpetuates the myth that certain foods can be combined to help you to lose weight. One unforeseen effect is that some people follow the Hay diet principles by cutting back too much on carbohydrates. As a result, the proportion of fat in the diet can increase, leading to possible weight gain and health problems such as coronary heart disease.

Benefits
Despite the problems with the Hay diet's rationale, weight loss can be achieved by following this diet because of the reduction in fat and calories that results from restricting the range of foods allowed. The diet also encourages a healthy consumption of fruits and vegetables and a reduction in fat intake, which is in line with what nutritionists today recommend.

VERY LOW CALORIE DIET

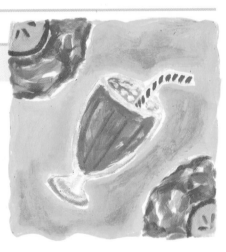

This diet became very popular in the early 1980s as a means of rapid weight loss. It is usually based around a flavoured milkshake or snack bar which supplies the recommended daily amount of vitamins, proteins, minerals and fat and up to 600 calories. Although satisfactory for short-term use (a few days), any weight lost is likely to be regained when normal eating habits are resumed. This diet is too severe for a long-term programme of weight control and does nothing to encourage healthy eating habits, which is essential if weight loss is to be maintained.

Rationale
This diet depends on the fact that if the body is given a low energy intake it is compelled to draw the additional energy it needs from fat stores: rapid weight loss will be inevitable. The problem is that the body becomes efficient at functioning on less energy, so the metabolic rate declines, and the body tends to use up lean tissue from muscles (including the heart) as well as fat.

Risks
Although temporary use of this type of diet is unlikely to cause harm, there is concern that in the long term it may present a risk to health. The Department of Health in the UK advises a limit of four weeks on this type of diet. Pregnant women, people with chronic health conditions, children and the elderly should never follow a diet so low in calories.

Benefits
Very low calorie meals are often complete in vitamins and mineral content whereas home cooked meals are often not. A more acceptable way of using the diet is as a replacement for just one or two of the smaller meals of the day, continuing with the normal main meal. In this way a diet of around 1000 calories a day can be achieved, with no danger to health.

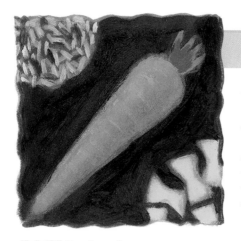

LOW-FAT DIET

A diet that recommends significantly lowering your total fat intake – by excluding or limiting foods that are particularly rich in fat such as fried food, many types of meat, condiments, dairy products and dressings – can be considered a low-fat diet. Usually a higher intake of carbohydrate foods, fruits and vegetables is suggested which will bring your diet more in line with healthy eating recommendations. Weight loss is usually successful on this diet and is likely to be maintained provided the low-fat eating principles are adopted on a permanent basis.

Rationale
The principle behind this diet is similar to that of the low carbohydrate diet (see page 104) in that avoidance of certain foods will lead to a reduction in total calories. This diet makes more sense as fat is the most concentrated source of energy, providing twice as many calories per gram as carbohydrate or protein. It is also the least satiating, and so the easiest to overconsume.

Risks
Some low-fat diets make misleading claims such as perpetuating the myth that cellulite is caused by toxic substances and that these diets help to spot-reduce fat. Many also propose a fat intake below the minimum recommendation of 30 g (1oz) a day. Some fat is required to absorb fat soluble vitamins and provide essential fatty acids which the body cannot make.

Benefits
Currently, people tend to eat far more fat than they need and low-fat diets can be used to bring fat intake down to the recommended level. Reducing fat intake in the diet is proven to reduce risks of heart disease. The other advantage is that this diet is easy to maintain – starchy foods add bulk to the diet and are more filling. Eating habits may also change for the better.

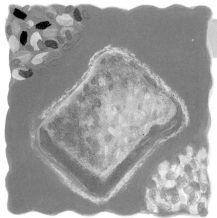

HIGH-FIBRE DIET

This diet recommends a high intake of fibre from sources such as fruits, vegetables, cereals, nuts and wholefoods. Provided this means a reduction in daily calorie intake, a high-fibre diet can result in weight loss. It is important to choose a diet that suggests a balanced range of food to ensure the body receives all the nutrients, vitamins and minerals essential for health. Fibre intake should not exceed 18 g per day as this level can interfere with the body's mineral supply. Remember that there is a difference between soluble and insoluble fibre – you need both for a balanced diet. The former can even help counteract some of the latter's negative effects.

Rationale
A high-fibre regimen can aid weight loss by increasing the bulk of the diet, rapidly giving a sensation of 'fullness' on fewer calories. This principle forms the basis of many popular diets. Fibre is vital to health. Insoluble fibre (in rice, bran and nuts) aids digestion and is highly satiating, while soluble fibre (in bread, pulses, fruits and vegetables) can help lower cholesterol.

Risks
The amount of fibre often recommended is very high and may produce side effects such as flatulence and diarrhoea. People with irritable bowel syndrome (IBS) may also find that their condition is exacerbated. A large intake of bran can bind minerals such as iron and zinc and prevent their absorption by the body, although soluble fibre can increase absorption.

Benefits
Most nutritionists agree that a high fibre intake is beneficial, particularly in the form of cereals, legumes (beans and pulses), fruits and vegetables. It can help to reduce the risk of some kinds of cancer, particularly cancer of the colon, and also helps prevent other gut problems, like diverticulosis. The decrease in fat that often results from following this diet is a bonus.

VEGETARIAN DIET

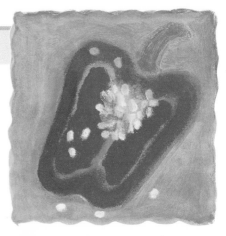

This diet excludes animal flesh and products. A vegan diet also excludes all animal by-products such as milk and other dairy items, eggs and perhaps even honey. In order to lose weight, total calorie intake must be reduced but vegetarian diets can rely heavily on dairy products, so vegetarians need to be careful to choose low-fat varieties. Cutting out meat is helpful for reducing saturated fats and cholesterol intake, but meat is an important source of iron, B_{12} and zinc. These nutrients must be replaced by other foods in the diet – a good variety of grains and pulses can provide missing nutrients – or it may be necessary to take a vitamin or mineral supplement.

Rationale

The theory of vegetarianism when practised for healthy eating is that the low amount of fat and animal protein consumed will be easier for the digestion, aid liver functioning and detoxify the body. As the diet is high in fruit and vegetables which are low in calories, weight loss is usually possible but it is also important to keep a check on fat for a lower total calorie intake.

Risks

Vegans should eat foods fortified with vitamin B_{12} as this can only be found naturally in animal products. Another area of concern for vegans and vegetarians is not getting enough iron and zinc from their diet and sometimes calcium. They must also make sure they receive a wide range of proteins from foods such as beans and pulses, nuts, bread, rice, pasta and potatoes.

Benefits

A well-planned vegetarian diet is an excellent way to learn healthy eating habits. An emphasis on wholegrain cereals, pulses, potatoes or rice will ensure a good intake of fibre, iron and the B vitamins (except B_{12}). The exclusion of meat and, for vegans, dairy products, will dramatically reduce fat in the diet, lowering the risk of many diseases including heart disease.

CALORIE-COUNTED DIET

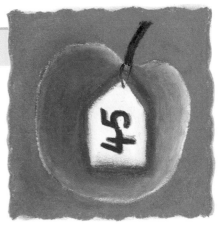

This diet involves weighing and assessing the calorie content of food items in order to regulate intake of total calories at a low enough level to produce weight loss. It can be extremely difficult to weigh food accurately and mistakes can be made in calculating total calorie intake. Frequently people stop weighing food after a few days, and over time portion sizes increase, calorie intake creeps up and the rate of weight loss therefore declines. Some people can also become unduly preoccupied with calorie counting, losing sight of equally important nutritional considerations like fat content.

Rationale

This diet restricts energy intake by counting calories, thus all types of foods are permitted provided a certain calorie limit is not exceeded. If this limit is below the individual energy requirement, weight will be lost. Almost all diets are based on some form of energy restriction, although many come disguised as 'magic' formulas making false nutritional claims.

Risks

Avoid calorie-counting diets that omit some food groups while emphasising others and those that do not properly balance nutrient intake. These can of course be tailored to better standards but some people may lack the nutritional knowledge to make adequate choices. When allowed to select their own diet by counting calories, some people will select unhealthy foods.

Benefits

This type of diet is popular as it does not require any food restrictions and can be adapted to suit individual needs and taste. The diet can promote good eating habits by education, as you learn how much foods vary in their calorie content and how to tailor your food shopping towards low calorie options. Try to check fat content as well as keeping down calories.

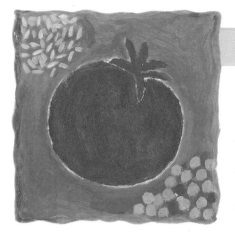

THE PRITIKIN DIET

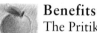

Developed in the 1970s by Nathan Pritikin, this diet is characteristically high in unrefined, complex carbohydrate foods, primarily wholegrains, vegetables and fruits, and very low in meat and animal by-products (and protein in general), caffeine, fat, cholesterol, sugar and salt. Nathan Pritikin was originally an engineer and inventor in the Second World War who designed and manufactured army munitions. After developing heart problems he became interested in diet and health and developed a programme to re-educate people into healthy eating in order to combat the threat of heart disease.

Rationale
Pritikin's approach combined diet and exercise programmes designed to promote fitness, reduce weight and lengthen life. He believed that a drastic reduction in fat (to less than 10 per cent of the total calories) and severe restrictions in sugar or honey, caffeine, cholesterol, salt and alcohol should have beneficial effects on the body and significantly reduce the risk of heart disease.

Risks

The bulk of the Pritikin diet is derived from vegetables, so protein and fat intake can be below the recommended daily amounts. The rigidity of the diet makes it difficult to stick to and therefore unlikely to change people's eating habits, which is vital for long-term weight maintenance. Cutting out all dairy products also restricts the amount of calcium in the diet.

Benefits
The Pritikin diet includes a lot of sound advice, and particularly stresses the link between diet and exercise. The programmes have had good results for clients in Pritikin's Longevity Centre in California where significant improvements in blood cholesterol have been documented. But the same improvements can be achieved by following less restrictive diets.

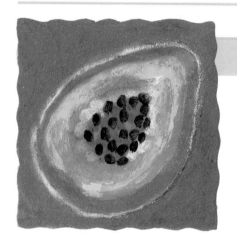

THE RAW ENERGY DIET

In this diet, foods that are processed or cooked in any way are excluded, and between 50 and 75 per cent of total calorie intake is from raw fruits, vegetables, nuts and seeds. An inventive array of salads and fruit desserts are recommended as well as no-cook soups, home-made yoghurt, nut loaves and raw cakes. The diet considerably lowers the fat intake and calorie count and is therefore a successful diet for weight loss. However, it is difficult to consistently prepare food from raw ingredients and can be time consuming. Some of the ideas can be incorporated into simpler healthy eating plans.

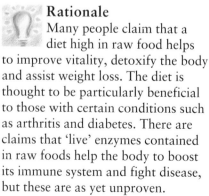

Rationale
Many people claim that a diet high in raw food helps to improve vitality, detoxify the body and assist weight loss. The diet is thought to be particularly beneficial to those with certain conditions such as arthritis and diabetes. There are claims that 'live' enzymes contained in raw foods help the body to boost its immune system and fight disease, but these are as yet unproven.

Risks

This diet may be deficient in some nutrients such as iron and vitamin B_{12} which are abundant in animal foods. Taken to extremes over a long period, the diet may also lead to other micro-nutrient deficiencies. If too little fat is eaten, the intake and absorption of fat soluble vitamins may be inadequate. The diet is unsuitable for children, pregnant women and the elderly.

Benefits

Eating a diet based on fruits and vegetables does provide the body with plenty of fibre and many nutrients, particularly beta-carotene, vitamin C and potassium. The raw food diet has a low energy density which can be useful for a weight loss programme as it helps to suppress appetite, and means you can fill up without taking in too many calories.

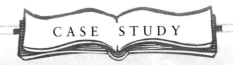

The Yo-yo Dieter

Yo-yo dieters constantly try to achieve their ideal weight by dieting. They typically spend several months of each year following a weight-reducing diet, with periods of normal eating in between. Unfortunately, many people find that the weight is quickly regained when they come off the diet and so they begin a continuous cycle of weight loss and weight gain.

Alison is a 26-year-old hairdresser who recently got married. She has never been slim and has always had a sweet tooth. She dieted in preparation for her wedding to David and lost 15 kg (2 st 5 lb), reaching 60 kg (9 st 6 lb), a healthy weight for her height. Married life suited Alison and as a result her eating habits became very relaxed again. After six months she was back to her original weight, but as her holiday approached she decided to diet again and lost 10 kg (1 st 8 lb). On her return her weight crept up and she soon weighed 70 kg (11 stone). Alison realises that this pattern of weight fluctuation is likely to continue throughout her life unless she makes permanent changes.

WHAT SHOULD ALISON DO?

Alison should start by keeping a food diary of everything she eats, for at least two weeks. A diary often helps to highlight where a person is going wrong and can be useful when discussing the problem with a partner or health professional. She should also identify ways of improving her diet. For instance, she should try to avoid skipping lunch which usually means she eats a chocolate bar or biscuits in the afternoon to keep her going. A sandwich would be much less harmful to her weight and more beneficial to her health. It is also important for Alison to think about a long-term exercise programme as this will help to increase her energy expenditure and overall fitness.

Action Plan

FITNESS
Begin a regular exercise programme to help to keep weight down and to provide a distraction from snacks and sweets.

EATING HABITS
Choose high-fibre foods for lunch such as baked potatoes or a home-made soup which can be frozen for use later on. Substitute fruit for high-fat snacks.

FAMILY
Talk to David about the need for support and ask if he would be willing to join her in some form of exercise.

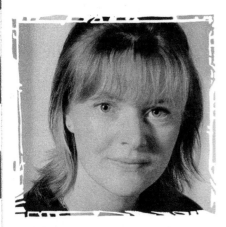

FITNESS
Lack of exercise makes it difficult to reduce or stabilise weight.

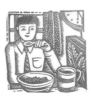

EATING HABITS
Irregular eating habits can lead to someone having high fat or sugary snacks in place of low-calorie foods.

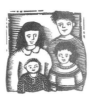

FAMILY
Partners play an important role in offering practical and emotional support when a person is trying to regulate his or her weight.

HOW THINGS TURNED OUT FOR ALISON

Alison now structures her daily meals and has stopped snacking. She cycles 7 km (4 miles) to work every day and as a result her fitness has increased dramatically, helping her to lose 7 kg (1 stone). She has given up chocolate, apart from the odd treat, and always has lunch instead of snacking on biscuits in the afternoon. She does not think that she will ever be thin but is happy that her weight is now stable and within the healthy range for her height.

DIETING AIDS AND GIMMICKS

The types of so-called weight-loss aids available today range from special foods for slimmers to pills, creams and patches. Unfortunately, few of these seem to be of genuine value.

Health stores, diet clinics and even your local supermarket may now have quick slimming aids on offer. You should think carefully before turning to dieting aids, however: first to determine if you do actually need to lose weight, and second to decide whether the diet aid is going to help. Many are of very little value and some can even be dangerous.

DIET BOOKS

For many people, purchase of a diet book is the first step in their weight-loss project. Often people turn to new diets because old ones have failed. New diet books are always appearing, but few deliver an entirely new concept. Diets only work if they restrict energy intake, although from the nutritional point of view some are clearly better than others. Diet books that encourage rapid weight loss or allow only a limited selection of foods should be avoided. Many diet books don't give helpful advice on who needs to lose weight. They present the ideal body shape as that dictated by the fashion industry and often encourage people who are already a healthy weight to slim. The myth that cellulite is a special kind of fat that is caused by accumulating toxins also encourages some women of normal weight to restrict their intake of certain foods.

A good diet book can be a real help, however, both in terms of practical advice and inspiration. It should help you to establish whether or not you need to lose weight and advise a regime in line with dietary recommendations. Severe food restrictions are unnecessary and you should aim for a weight loss of 0.5–1 kg (1–2 lb) a week.

SPECIAL DIET FOODS

Meal replacements (see left) are becoming increasingly popular together with other low-calorie foods and slimming aids. In the UK, it is illegal to make claims for weight reduction unless the product specifies that weight loss can only occur 'as part of a calorie-controlled diet'. These products can be high in fat and sugar and they only work because total calorie intake is restricted by dramatically reducing food intake. Meal replacements usually make claims for rapid weight loss but do nothing to change eating habits. This means that as soon as you start eating your normal diet any weight lost is likely to be regained, and therefore they are

---

MEAL REPLACEMENTS

Meal replacements, usually bars or milkshakes, are meant to replace breakfast, lunch or both, providing all the vitamins and minerals essential to health. But no laws exist to control nutritional quality and some meals don't provide enough protein and fibre. Some people find that a gradual introduction to meal replacements helps them adjust to eating less. Meal replacements have increased dramatically in popularity with sales in the UK rising by 500 per cent since 1990.

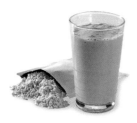

A MEAL IN A SHAKE
Although meal replacements can be useful in a calorie-controlled diet, they are only ever a short-term solution and do nothing to encourage healthy eating habits.

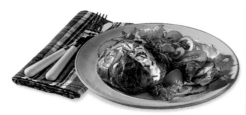

REAL FOOD ALTERNATIVES
The calorie content of light meals – such as this baked potato with cottage cheese and salad – is about the same as a meal replacement but will fill you up much more.

unsuitable for long-term use. Another drawback is cost – it is much cheaper to go on an ordinary reduced calorie diet than to buy meal replacements. Many health food shops also sell herbal supplements which claim to promote fast, effective weight loss. These usually contain various plant substances such as lecithin, kelp or spirulina, ginseng, ginger and tea. Their effects have never been proved in scientific experiments.

GIMMICKS

The diet industry is constantly launching new slimming 'aids'. Some are gadgets: special clothing to wear which claims to increase your metabolic rate, and massage machines and electric pads which are supposed to exercise your muscles by contracting them. Other gimmicks such as diet creams and body wraps have become popular despite the fact that, as with all slimming gimmicks, there is no evidence that they work in the long-term. Some, such as weight-loss patches, can even be dangerous.

Diet creams

These have been invented to target cellulite, despite the fact that experts insist cellulite is just normal fat. It is suggested that fat cells beneath the skin 'disintegrate' when the cream is rubbed onto the affected area, although scientific evidence does not support this claim. These creams may contain substances which cause a local increase in blood flow which causes the skin to tighten slightly thus improving its 'look'. However, they do not reduce the amount of fat present and even the slight 'firmness' of the skin that occurs with the massaging action is short term and will disappear when you stop using the cream.

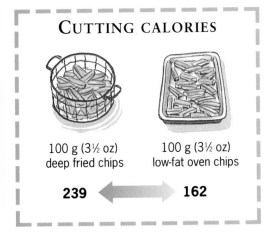

CUTTING CALORIES

100 g (3½ oz) deep fried chips

100 g (3½ oz) low-fat oven chips

239 ← → **162**

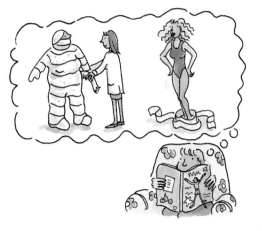

HOLD ON TO REALITY!
Treatments such as body wraps cannot perform miracles. Reaching ideal body weight is a long-term commitment and there really is no replacement for eating healthily and increasing your level of physical activity. Use special treatments to reward yourself for successful weight loss.

Body wraps – the easy way out?

Body wraps have become fashionable in many health farms and clinics as an easy way to lose weight. This usually entails being covered with mud and then wrapped in bandages. The theory is to open up the pores of the skin and draw out the toxins from the fat beneath. In fact, any reduction in weight is due to water loss through sweating and is quickly replenished by drinking fluids. The idea that some fat deposition is due to toxins has no scientific basis.

Weight-loss patches

Weight-loss patches promise to increase your metabolism by passing substances such as iodine into the bloodstream. Iodine is a mineral needed by the body to make thyroid hormone and is essential for controlling the rate of metabolism. But although the metabolic rate decreases if iodine is deficient in the diet, it cannot be increased by taking extra iodine and in any case, iodine deficiency is very rare in Britain. The amount of iodine that is present in skin patches is usually too small to have any effect. Thyroid hormone preparations do increase the metabolic rate, but in people with normal thyroid function they have a range of adverse effects including loss of muscle tissue and heart problems, and are not suitable as an aid to weight loss.

DIETING PILLS

The race to find a magic cure that dissolves fat away effortlessly has prompted research into 'miracle pills'. At best they are harmless, containing 'natural' herbal ingredients or vitamins which have no effect; at worst they can cause dangerous side effects such as nausea, high blood pressure, insomnia and even hallucinations.

New diet pills are advertised in the press all the time, some claiming 'breakthrough' scientific discoveries. Most of these claims are unsubstantiated by modern science.

There are various classes of drugs and 'natural' products used to treat obesity and they work in different ways. For example, diuretics remove water from the body by prompting urination, thus weight loss is quick but this is water and not fat and is quickly regained. Caffeine and many herbal mixtures may also act as diuretics. Bulking agents present in many diet pills claim to make you feel full quicker if you take them just before meals. These include natural forms of fibre such as guar gum and sugar beet fibre. If taken in large amounts these can cause intestinal blockages but most contain amounts too small to have any effect.

Many over-the-counter preparations used to treat asthma or hay fever contain theophylline and ephedrine – two drugs that are known to increase the metabolic rate. Theophylline is related to caffeine and is present in various plants such as tea, coffee, cocoa and the cola plant. Ephedrine is also a naturally occurring drug that has been used in medicine for thousands of years. Preparations containing ephedrine have been used in China for at least 5000 years under the name of 'ma huang'. However, clinical trials to assess the effectiveness of these drugs in the treatment of obesity are lacking. Large doses can have unpleasant side effects such as nausea and high blood pressure. Guarana, which has recently been approved for use in the UK, also contains compounds that are related to caffeine. There are many other substances which claim to burn fat and are sold over the counter at inflated prices. These include L-carnitine, chromium picolinate, hydroxycitric acid, choline and inositol. There is no scientific evidence to suggest that any of these affect weight loss.

Prescription drugs

A number of prescription drugs can cause weight loss. Some such as amphetamines and related compounds, however, have side effects and are potentially addictive. There has been concern within the health industry that some diet clinics may be too quick to dispense these types of drugs, sometimes even to people who already have a healthy body weight. It is unwise to attend a diet clinic or take any drugs or diet pills without checking their validity with your family doctor first.

A very limited number of drugs are available on prescription to obese people for the purpose of losing weight, usually only if their health is endangered by their weight. These are not miracle cures, but they are safe and used in conjunction with a sensible eating plan can help people to lose a little extra weight. But clinical trials show that weight loss generally only continues for about six months, and weight is often regained when treatment is stopped.

The pharmaceutical industry is always searching for new drugs for obesity, but it is increasingly recognised that there is unlikely to be a miracle cure which promotes weight loss without effort. Drugs will help to reinforce and maximise weight loss achieved by changes in diet and lifestyle.

SPOT REDUCTION

Many popular diets provide detailed advice on how to slim down parts of the body, particularly the hips and thighs. This is, unfortunately, another myth: it is not possible to spot reduce fat except by liposuction, a surgical technique which removes fat from beneath the skin by aspirating it through a needle. Liposuction can have unpleasant side effects and leave permanent scars and some studies suggest that fat which is removed may be quickly replaced.

Body shape and fat deposition are mostly genetically determined and weight loss cannot be targeted to a particular part of your body. When you go on a diet fat is first lost from the abdominal cavity, shoulders and face, and then the hips and thighs. Exercise, however, can alter body shape by improving muscle tone and should be an integral part of any weight-loss plan that is designed for long-term success.

TREAT YOURSELF
Massage can improve the circulation, helping to tone skin and muscle, but it cannot actually produce weight loss. Its main benefit lies in relaxing the body and enhancing general mental well-being; essential for a healthy lifestyle and maintaining the motivation needed for dieting.

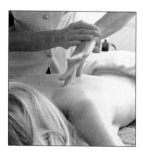

JOINING A WEIGHT-LOSS GROUP

Diet groups have helped millions of overweight people lose weight successfully. Many experts agree that they offer some of the best techniques to help you to lose weight and keep it off.

Diet books and isolated weight-loss programmes lack the help and support which comes through contact with other people going through a similar ordeal. Slimmers are also exposed to role models who have managed to lose weight and keep it off by changing their lifestyle.

CHOOSING A GROUP

There are many weight-loss groups to choose from – some are listed in your local directory, or alternatively your doctor may be able to offer useful advice. Diet groups are not for everyone and the best way to find out if it suits you is to attend a couple of meetings and see for yourself. Large commercial diet clubs such as Weight Watchers, Slimming Clubs, Rosemary Conley and Jenny Craig are among the best-known in the business, but there are also plenty of non-profit community groups to choose from, some run by local dietitians.

Commercial clubs usually charge a fee to join and then weekly meeting fees. For your money, you receive a diet and exercise plan, private weigh-in each week and group talks on how to improve eating habits. Personal attention is available for those who need it. Diet plans can vary, but many clubs offer sound nutritional advice with an emphasis on low-fat, high-carbohydrate diets. Another positive aspect is that they do not encourage rapid weight loss. A study published in the *Lancet* in 1990, testing the efficacy of various diets in overweight individuals, found slimming clubs among the most successful methods of losing weight.

continued on page 116

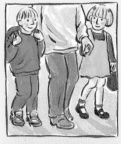

QUICK FITNESS TIP
Try to avoid taking unnecessary trips in the car. Instead, walk whenever possible, such as when taking the children to school or shopping locally.

LIFE ON A HEALTH FARM

Health farms, spas and weekend clinics provide luxurious surroundings where people can detoxify or lose weight. They are removed from the distractions of everyday life, and guests are encouraged to exercise, eat sensibly and relax.

Services such as exercise classes, massage, sauna, hydrotherapy, dietitians, lectures, beauty therapy, osteopathy, reflexology and aromatherapy are all available, together with sport and leisure activities like riding or golf.

Guests may get a medical consultation to work out their best programme, and by the time they leave they will have learnt about and experienced lifestyle changes they can adopt permanently.

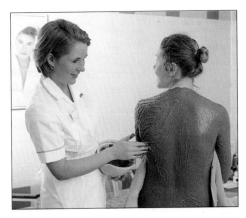

BEAUTY IS SKIN DEEP
Seaweed beauty treatments cleanse the skin, enhance the body's appearance and lull the guest into a relaxed state of mind.

113

Slimming Club Leader

For people who are concerned about being overweight but find it hard to stick to a diet, the informal, supportive environment of a slimming club can offer the encouragement they need to reach and maintain a healthy weight.

Origins

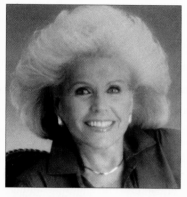

WEIGHT WATCHER PIONEER
Founder of Weight Watchers, Jean Nidetch could never have predicted its huge and lasting success. In the UK alone, around 230 000 members attend meetings each week.

By age 38, Jean Nidetch weighed 97 kg (15¼ stone) but secretly despised her condition. She soothed her low self-esteem with cycles of overeating and crash dieting. In 1961 she began attending an Obesity Clinic, and, following a low-cholesterol, calorie-controlled diet, attained a sustainable weight of 64 kg (10 stone). She linked her success with being able to talk over her problems with friends each week and the recognition of how emotional problems can lead to unhealthy eating habits. In 1963 she founded Weight Watchers in New York to help others to achieve similar results.

A commercial slimming club leader is simply a successful slimmer who has been trained to coordinate and conduct the weekly weight-loss meetings on behalf of the slimming organisation. To qualify for training they will have completed a successful weight-loss programme with the organisation and then successfully maintained their target weight. Thus the group leader provides a positive role model who understands the whole experience of being overweight and changing their lifestyle to lose that weight. The leader's training covers basic principles of psychology and health, as well as more advanced skills of behaviour modification and group interaction and communication. They learn how to guide and motivate group members to maintain and produce lifestyle changes of their own.

How do I join a slimming club?

The parent organisation of your chosen club can tell you where the nearest meeting centre is. Meetings are usually held weekly and you should have no trouble finding a time to suit you. Then simply go along and register.

What happens at group meetings?

The leader will register your membership (although with some clubs you don't have to join until after the first meeting), introduce you to fellow group members and weigh you. Your weight is confidential, and remains so throughout the

programme. Sessions centre around a group discussion of the issues and problems surrounding weight loss and dieting. Group leaders use their training to coordinate and guide the discussion, as well as teaching behavioural techniques to help members reform their eating habits. Although members do tend to discuss how they are doing with each other, confidentiality about your actual weight and the amounts lost will be observed at all times.

Every week your weight loss progress is checked and group members discuss their own progress and problems, talk about their methods and exchange advice. The leader will provide support and advice on aspects of nutrition and exercise. You may even have demonstrations of calorie-controlled recipes or slimming products, possibly with pressure to buy.

How do I know how much weight to lose?

Setting realistic goals and a sensible personal agenda for weight loss is an extremely important step and your slimming club will give you as much guidance as possible. The group leader will have charts and tables which are used to work out your ideal healthy weight range, but you set your own targets. This means you can choose to lose as little as 3 kg (6 lb 8 oz) or as much as you need to reach your ideal weight – the club will support whatever you decide as long as your weight goal is within the healthy range for your height.

How do I actually lose weight in a slimming club?

Many clubs work on a points system. They provide comprehensive food lists and tables where a score is allocated to various foodstuffs, based on their calorific value. You are allotted a points budget for each day, which is based on your age, sex, starting weight and activity levels. The budget is set at a level that will ensure that your calorie expenditure exceeds your intake. Within this budget you are free to eat whatever you like (although healthy eating guidelines, such as lowering levels of fat and cholesterol, should also be considered). There may even be a list of very low-calorie foods, of which you can eat unlimited amounts. You will have to keep a record of what you've eaten, so that your points tally can be calculated. In some cases, points can be 'saved' for special occasions or 'earned' through exercise. The basic theme of the weight control plan is to eat a diet that is balanced and full of variety.

Do I have to exercise?

Different clubs have different philosophies towards exercise. Most will encourage you to become more active, but few actually include exercise routines as part of the weekly sessions. In most clubs, you can earn points by doing exercise.

Can anyone join?

People under 16 will need permission from their doctor. People whose Body Mass Index shows that they are underweight will not be allowed to join, and anyone with a health condition should obtain their doctor's consent before starting a slimming programme.

How long do most weight loss programmes last?

Obviously this will depend on how much weight you aim to lose and how well you manage to stick to the diet plan you are given. The maximum healthy weekly weight loss is between 0.5–1 kg (1–2 lb) per week. If you are losing more than this you should have a medical check-up and it may be necessary to come off the diet.

Do organisations provide support to people who have reached their target weight?

Yes. To help you maintain your weight loss you will be welcome to continue attending meetings, perhaps even free of charge (where you can help motivate others). Alternatively, you may be given a programme to take home that contains advice on how to maintain your new weight.

Are there any regulatory bodies for these slimming clubs?

There is no official regulatory body, but any weight loss claims made in advertisements or promotional literature are bound by the Advertising Standards Authority's regulations. Reputable slimming organisations prepare their diets and food plans along the government's guidelines on nutrition, diet and weight control.

WHAT YOU CAN DO AT HOME

It is a good idea to supplement your membership of a slimming club with a home exercise programme. As most clubs don't include exercise in their weight plans, following your own programme will help you to consolidate your achievements in the class, and can even earn you 'points' for your calorie budget. Some people find exercise videos helpful, particularly if they have never attended formal exercise classes, or are worried about exercising in the company of others. You can perform aerobic exercises in the privacy of your own living room, and take things at your own pace. Following exercises on screen can help you come to grips with them; you can replay movements that you find difficult until you've mastered them. Making up your own exercises is not advisable. All the exercises chosen for home workouts will be easy to copy without risk of injury. A good video will start with a series of warm-up exercises before moving on to a comprehensive programme that works all the major muscle groups, without risking strains or sprains. To ensure this, be careful to select a video that advertises approval by a government body or well-known and respected health and fitness organisation.

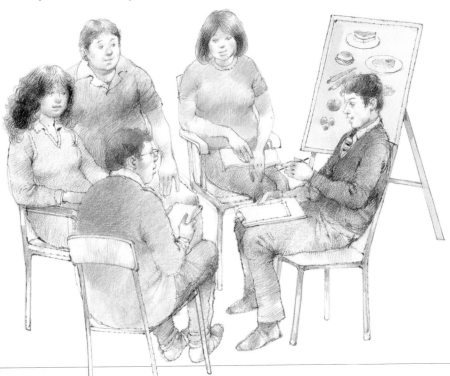

PRIVATE CLINICS

Some private slimming clinics both in the UK and abroad still prescribe potentially addictive drugs to slimmers. You should never take amphetamine derivatives. Many individuals who attend private slimming clinics are only mildly overweight or do not need to lose weight at all. It is worth asking your doctor's advice first if you are thinking of attending such a clinic.

HEALTH CLUBS

Some slimmers find health clubs that emphasise physical activity helpful. Most provide the necessary advice and support for people at all levels of fitness and there is a wide range of activities to choose from. Weight training, gym workouts, aerobic classes and swimming can all have a positive effect on the mind and the body. There is considerable evidence that an increased level of physical activity is one of the best ways to prevent weight gain, especially after a period of successful weight loss, but it is difficult to lose weight through exercise alone without changing your diet. Unfortunately, many health clubs do not provide qualified dietary advice to members. Another drawback is that health clubs can be quite expensive. Look for those that offer special rates at off-peak times.

HEALTH FARMS

There are now many health farms which offer you the chance to relax in a pleasant environment that is equipped with everything necessary for relaxation and weight loss. Healthy, balanced meals, exercise programmes and health treatments such as massage are provided and many see this as a welcome break from the stresses of everyday living. However, health farms are a very expensive way to lose weight and there is no guarantee that a short stay in this environment will be enough to enable you to change the bad habits of a lifetime.

BEHAVIOUR THERAPY GROUPS

For most overweight individuals, psychological factors associated with obesity have to be overcome to ensure successful weight loss. Food is used by many to cope with the boredom, loneliness, insecurity and frustration which are a part of life. Old habits are difficult to change, but many weight-loss groups now use behavioural therapy to try to change eating habits. Large slimming organisations such as Weight Watchers also use elements of standard behavioural modification techniques in their programmes. People who try behaviour modification on their own and fail may benefit from group therapy, but it is worth checking the credentials of the professionals involved in any programme. Some group leaders do not have adequate qualifications. If in doubt, your doctor or dietitian can suggest a suitable behaviour modification centre.

The aim of behaviour therapy is to help people identify negative factors which encourage bad eating habits and replace these with new patterns of behaviour. Slimmers are encouraged to keep food and activity diaries, remove foods that may precipitate binge eating from the home and work environment, and pay more attention to the act of eating. Once the pitfalls have been identified, a programme can be adapted to suit individual needs. Slimmers are taught to reward themselves for positive behaviour, rather than weight loss.

Being with other people in a similar situation can also have a positive impact on behaviour. The success of any programme depends on the skill and experience of the therapist, as well as individual motivation. Weight loss can only occur if the slimmer follows a calorie-restricted diet, although changing behaviour can enhance motivation and help to make this easier to achieve.

Some weight-loss groups are also employing meditation techniques or hypnosis to try and change eating habits. These methods may help people relax and deal positively with everyday tensions that induce overeating, provided they are carried out by trained specialists. However, there is no concrete proof that these techniques induce significant weight loss. Adequate dietary advice is crucial to long-term success in any weight-loss group using behaviour therapy.

There is an argument that behavioural methods should be applied to the whole family, not just the overweight individual. Studies have shown that weight loss is more likely if spouses of subjects participate actively in treatment. However, it is important to consider all the options available before joining a particular weight-loss group. Any treatment offered that is not based on sound nutritional principles is unlikely to work in the long term.

STEP-BY-STEP FITNESS
Joining a health club or an aerobics class may be an expense, but the professional guidance will help you to avoid injury and get the most out of your time. It will also provide ongoing support and increase your motivation.

CHAPTER 8

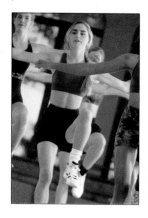

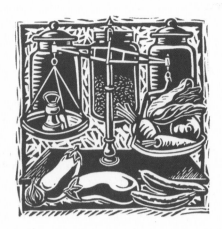

YOUR WEIGHT-CONTROL PLAN

The secret of a successful weight-control plan is to tailor your diet and exercise regimes to suit your own needs. This means looking at your lifestyle both at home and at work, and setting realistic goals which take account of the existing demands on your time and energy.

STARTING A WEIGHT-CONTROL PROGRAMME

If it is to be successful, a weight-control programme needs to be introduced with care, setting a realistic long-term goal and establishing ways to keep yourself motivated.

Earlier chapters have discussed the extent to which people's ideas of 'ideal' weight are shaped by outside forces: advertising and the media set goals which are impossible for most people to attain. If your goal is to end up with the same statistics as a catwalk model you are probably destined to be disappointed. It is enlightening to realise that this body shape is natural for only 5 per cent of the population.

Your ideal weight should be based on a combination of your age, body mass index (BMI) and body shape. Once you establish which body shape you are you can form a more reasonable ideal weight goal.

FINDING YOUR IDEAL WEIGHT

If you are an endomorph or a mesomorph (see box, below) you will need to accept that your natural body shape is more rounded, and that basing a weight-control plan on the tall, thin body image of a fashion model – the typical ectomorph – will not be very helpful. Fixing your sights on this body image is likely to lead to a constant weight battle that is ultimately doomed to failure. It's more helpful to focus on a role model, such as an actor, TV presenter or show-business celebrity, who is closer to your own height and build, and who has a figure that you admire.

KNOWING YOUR BODY SHAPE

Most people fall into one of three body types: endomorphs, mesomorphs or ectomorphs. Establishing your body shape will help you to develop an exercise plan that targets the areas where you are most likely to put on weight. While you can't change where your body type distributes fat, you can firm up the muscles in the problem areas to give you more tone and shape.

Endomorphs should target the abdominal muscles to tone the stomach, while mesomorphs (the category most women fall into) should target the thighs and buttocks. The tall, slim ectomorphs should ensure their regime pays equal attention to all major muscle groups.

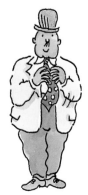

ENDOMORPHS (APPLE-SHAPED PEOPLE)
These people tend to put on weight around their stomachs and waists. Their legs tend to be shorter than their torsos and they are shorter in stature than the average.

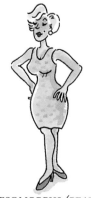

MESOMORPHS (PEAR-SHAPED PEOPLE)
Mesomorphs have hips wider than their shoulders and legs that are about the same length as their torsos. Weight is usually gained around the thighs, then hips and buttocks.

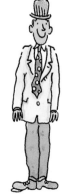

ECTOMORPHS (BEAN-POLE SHAPED PEOPLE)
They are taller with long legs in proportion to their torsos. Any excess weight is usually evenly distributed over the body. Most fashion models are ectomorphs.

Achieving your goals

Before embarking on your weight plan you need to accept that results are not going to be instantaneous. Successful, long-term weight loss results from gradual change that can be maintained over a long period of time; not crash diets that bring about only temporary weight loss. Your goal will best be achieved by re-orientating yourself to new ways of eating and exercising that you can practise for the rest of your life. First, however, you will need to prepare yourself for the changes that this new approach will bring to your everyday life.

Your lifestyle and needs

Remember that your ideal weight should take into account the demands that your lifestyle places on you. If you lead a particularly active life – for example, if you are a teacher chasing after young children all day – you need to recognise that your body needs more energy than a sedentary office worker to maintain effective functioning. However, even a sedentary person needs energy to function effectively. A weight-control plan should never mean starving yourself – but rather changing the main types of food you eat.

Until now you may have taken a large proportion of your energy as high-fat foods, and in addition eaten sweets, chocolate bars, or biscuits that are high in fat and sugar in order to give yourself a short-term energy boost. Instead you should aim to reduce your fat and sugar intake gradually and to increase the percentage of complex carbohydrate foods in your diet. Such foods, which include bread, rice and pasta, provide energy in a less concentrated form than fat but the energy is more slowly released in the body than that from simple sugar. This means the energy is more readily accessible and will also sustain you for longer periods.

WHICH DIET IF ANY?

Deciding to begin a weight-control programme doesn't necessarily mean deciding to begin a diet. The word itself conjures up images of lettuce leaves, carrots and starvation. In fact some studies suggest that strict dieting can encourage people to be obsessive about food, which may, in turn, lead to overeating. One study conducted in the United States in the 1950s examined 36 men who were put on a calorie-controlled diet that reduced their food intake by approximately half over a 12-week period. While all the men lost weight, it was observed that some members of the group became fixated on food to the point where they began to steal or hoard it. They also became depressed and apathetic. An examination of their eating habits after the period of dieting revealed a pattern of bingeing and loss of control over their eating habits.

Highly restrictive dieting can be counter-productive, and is not the best route to effective weight control. Successful weight control involves becoming better informed about foods, and particularly fat, so that your eating habits change permanently. When most people examine their current eating habits they find that a reduction could be made in the amount of fat and sugar eaten to reduce the total number of calories they consume each day. Making permanent changes to your eating habits and introducing regular exercise into your life will help you to lose weight, and can mean that you don't need to undertake more formalised diets, or reduce the volume of food you eat.

Some people, however, find that they need the discipline of a diet plan to keep them focused and motivated. Others need an initial sharp change in eating habits to introduce long-term change. If this is the case for you, make sure that you assess the benefits

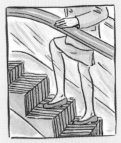

QUICK FITNESS TIP
Each time you use an escalator, walk up instead of letting the escalator do the leg work for you. Better still, use the stairs.

BURNING OFF CALORIES: *Rowing*

Rowing, either using a machine in the gym or a boat on water, is an excellent aerobic exercise. It puts all your body's major muscle groups to work and develops endurance.

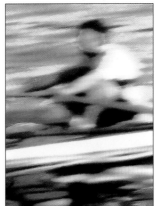

MUSCLE GROUPS BENEFITING
Rowing exercises muscles in your legs, chest, arms, abdomen, shoulders, back and buttocks.

EQUIPMENT
A sturdy rowing machine or you can hire a rowing boat.

CALORIES BURNT
During rowing, you expend an average of 11 calories per minute: that's 660 calories per hour.

A New Mother

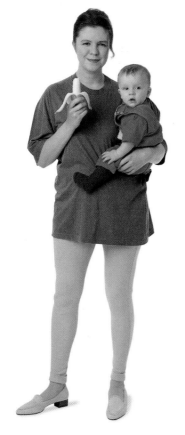

A young baby can quickly sabotage a new mother's well-laid plans for getting back to pre-pregnancy weight and shape. There are constant demands on time and energy, together with the exhausting effects of interrupted sleep. These make it hard to find the resources to exercise, or the will to prepare healthy meals. Convenience foods and snacks may be all you have time for or feel up to, with the result that you fail to shed the weight you put on during pregnancy and cannot regain your previous shape. Remember that your body has specific nutritional needs during breastfeeding and you should not diet during this time, but you can still begin a new healthy eating plan.

FOOD

PROBLEM 1
No time to cook proper meals
When you are rushed off your feet looking after a young baby, cooking proper meals may seem like a luxury. Instead you rely on convenience meals and processed food.

SOLUTION
Try to get a bit more support – friends, family and neighbours are often delighted to help so don't feel you have to do everything yourself. Use the extra time to prepare some healthy meals. Follow the basic rules of cutting down on fat and increasing fruit and vegetable intake. If your baby is eating solids you could liquidise your meal for baby to share. Remember that variety is a good way of ensuring that both you and your baby get all the nutrients you need.

PROBLEM 2
Sugary or high-fat snacks
Fatigue can leave you feeling lethargic, run-down and in need of an immediate energy boost from sweets and high-fat snacks.

SOLUTION
Turn snacking to your advantage. More, smaller meals each day may be better than a few large ones. Eat high fibre, low-fat, low-sugar snacks which will fill you up without adding too many calories. For an energy boost, eat a banana which is high in potassium, a mineral essential for muscle and nerve function; or try a handful of raisins which are high in iron but low in fat.

LIFESTYLE

PROBLEM 1
No time or energy to exercise
If you haven't kept up with your postnatal exercises your muscles won't have toned, and you will feel too tired to move on to aerobic exercise. Although a baby is a constant demand on your time, finding ways of exercising together can be stimulating for you both.

SOLUTION
Increasing activity levels will help you to get a net calorie loss, while toning exercises will tighten your muscles, improving your figure. Though you may feel too tired to do any exercise it is worth persevering, because in the long run your energy levels will increase. Involve your baby in your postnatal exercises; start by walking with your baby in a pram or a carrypack. Swimming is another aerobic exercise that you can both enjoy by joining a mother and baby class. Many pools also have child-minding facilities so that you can swim a few lengths on your own.

PROBLEM 2
Lack of sleep
The new baby disrupts your sleeping patterns, depleting your energy and leaving you tense and exhausted.

SOLUTION
Try practising some relaxation techniques whenever possible during the day. Meditation, visualisation or yoga can help your body recover from disrupted sleep and give you more energy.

CUTTING CALORIES

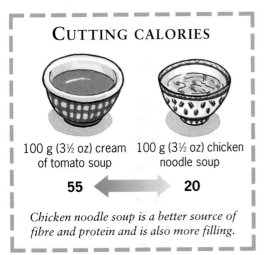

100 g (3½ oz) cream of tomato soup

100 g (3½ oz) chicken noodle soup

55 ⬅➡ **20**

Chicken noodle soup is a better source of fibre and protein and is also more filling.

before you start a diet to ensure you have made the right choice (see Chapter 7). Remember that a diet must follow sound nutritional guidelines by including all the major food groups and ensuring a plentiful intake of vital vitamins and minerals.

Carefully assess any published health risks and research any evidence about the diet's efficacy before you begin. Discuss your findings with your doctor so that together you can consider how the diet might affect you. It may be that the diet can be adapted slightly so that it suits your particular needs. Remember that for successful long-term weight management, diets should encourage healthier eating habits which can be continued after your target weight has been reached. Examine the technical demands of the diet, such as weighing food and counting calories, and ask yourself if you will be able to stick to it in the long term. Another important aspect to consider is whether the diet is within your budget and if you can successfully adapt your lifestyle to follow it.

Pathway to health

Natural therapies are of particular help if your eating habits are influenced by your emotions. Stress can play a major role in inducing bad diet habits like comfort eating and snacking on the run, which can be responsible for weight gain. Introducing relaxation programmes such as meditation or reflexology into your daily life (see Chapter 6) may help you to break the cycle of high fat snacking or bingeing.

For example, can it be worked in with your partner's eating habits, or your children's dietary needs?

Whatever dietary change you make, or whatever diet you follow, you should also consider introducing more exercise into your life. Most experts agree that exercise combined with diet provides the best results for long-term weight loss and maintenance of reduced weight (see Chapter 5).

The psychology of diets

Studies have shown that many dieters fail when an obsessive attitude is taken about following the diet. If you feel that you have blown the diet completely by eating one chocolate bar, you are more likely to start binge eating. Try to avoid becoming obsessive and forgive yourself for the odd slip up. It is difficult to always maintain rigid eating controls.

If you understand the principles of healthy eating and exercise, and realise that eating a three-course restaurant meal one night may mean smaller servings of food the next day, or a longer period of exercise, you will be able to master the eating challenges everyone faces from time to time. If your weight goal is to be achieved within a realistic period of time, one or two 'infringements' of the rules will have little fundamental effect. As long as you make the effort to return to your plan, and don't use occasional faltering as an excuse to give up, your goal will still be attainable.

MOTIVATION

Try to keep a positive outlook while you establish your weight-control plan. As well as keeping focused on your long-term goal, set yourself interim goals to aim for that are well within your abilities to achieve. For example, set a small target weight loss of 2.5 kg (5½ lb) after the first three weeks of your diet and exercise programme.

Set dietary goals too – aim to eat an extra piece of fruit each day or to stop taking sugar in tea and coffee. Small goals are important, because they help you to keep motivated even if weight loss seems slow. Any step in the right direction will help towards achieving long-term goals.

Be sure to praise yourself for all of your successes and to record them in a diary or notebook (see right) that you can refer to whenever you need a psychological boost.

RECORDING YOUR PROGRESS

Keeping a diary during your weight-management plan can help you to stay positive and determined. You may go through a week where you do not lose any weight at all, but can be spurred on by reminding yourself of your successes so far. The most obvious entry is your weekly weight readings but there are several other things you could record:

▶ *The results of the step test (see page 84).*

▶ *Your waist-hip ratio (see page 24).*

▶ *Positive feedback such as flattering comments regarding your appearance.*

▶ *Feelings of increased well-being.*

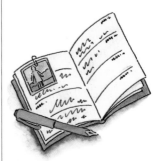

PHOTOGRAPHIC EVIDENCE
Include a photograph in your diary so that you can see how far you have come since you began your weight-control programme. See page 129 for how to set up a suitable snap shot.

Rather than focusing on weighing yourself obsessively, set exercise targets that you have to meet, and take pride in watching your fitness levels develop. As your fitness increases you will have the satisfaction of knowing that your muscles are being toned, your general health and vitality improving, and your metabolic rate increasing. All of these factors will improve your general appearance and you will feel an increased sense of well-being. These changes should prove that you are making progress.

Find ways to make food control fun

Try different healthy snacks to discover the ones you really enjoy, and make sure you turn to them when you feel the emotional need for comfort eating, rather than to high-fat or high-sugar snacks and sweets. This will help you to keep to your weight-control programme, and so be less likely to lapse during times of emotional crisis.

You should also adjust the way you view the dietary changes you have adopted so that they add fun and interest to your life, rather than making dieting seem like a chore. All good diet plans recommend including more fruit and vegetables into your daily meals, so try new produce, giving yourself the occasional exotic treat. For example try a new vegetable to liven up your main courses. Plantains might make a substitute for potatoes – they vary in flavour as they ripen, from potato to sweet potato to banana – and can be cooked in the same way as you would ordinary potatoes. Celeriac, or celery root, can be boiled, fried, stewed or used in salads.

There is also a whole range of unusual fruits that you could try for dessert or as a healthy snack. A custard apple or cherimoya has creamy, custard-flavoured flesh, and is a good source of potassium and vitamin C. Cape gooseberries have a piquant taste and are ideal for jam-making. Persimmon, a popular autumn fruit in the East, is increasingly available here under the name Sharon fruit and has a complex, sweet flavour. A selection of these fruits could be used together to make an exotic fruit salad.

INCREASING YOUR MOTIVATION

A weight-loss plan, built around a low-fat diet and regular exercise to improve your level of fitness, will lead to many health benefits as well as helping with weight loss. You will feel more energetic and healthy as you progress with your regime. You will also be lowering your risk of many chronic diseases including coronary heart disease and cancer. These are all important reasons for losing weight, but you may need other spurs to boost your determination, willpower and self-motivation.

▶ *Find a photograph of yourself when you were slimmer. Keep it prominently displayed as a reminder of what you can achieve.*

▶ *Find a partner in your plan, a friend who shares your long-term goal. Establish an exercise regime together, and share tips on recipes and low-fat shopping.*

▶ *Enlist your family's support: dieting will be much easier if they share in your new healthy eating, low-fat approach or at the very least don't undermine your efforts.*

▶ *Each time you chart considerable progress in weight loss or fitness, give yourself a reward: buy a new item of clothing or some flowers, or plan an outing to a favourite place.*

▶ *Keep exercise clothing and equipment around the house to remind you so that you don't slip up on sessions. Keeping your running shoes beside the bed, for example, can serve as a useful memory prod.*

▶ *Stop thinking negatively and instead focus your mind on the improvements that you have made so far. Start each day with a positive affirmation or two such as 'today I will eat well, feel great and look better than ever'. This is called autosuggestion (see page 97) and can go a long way towards improving your self-esteem and motivation.*

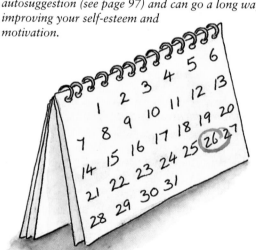

SETTING A TARGET DATE TO AIM FOR
Set down the date of an event or engagement to provide you with a weight-loss goal to work towards: something that is not unrealistically soon, but is four or five months away, and that is important to you. Perhaps a special holiday that you want to be fit and healthy for or a friend's wedding.

A Retired Person

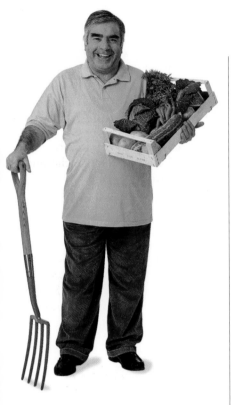

FOOD

PROBLEM 1
Slower metabolism leads to weight gain

Because the body's metabolic rate declines with age, people can gain weight if they don't reduce the amount of food that they eat.

SOLUTION

Try to reduce the size of your portions gradually, and change the balance of your meals to more filling complex carbohydrate-based meals to help you feel satiated. For example, starting the day with porridge and increasing the intake of rice, potatoes and bread with meals, will help you feel full and eat less.

PROBLEM 2
Less money to spend on food

For many people retirement can mean less to spend on food, leading to buying more high-fat processed foods. Reduced mobility can also affect the types of foods bought.

SOLUTION

Eating low-fat and nutritious food doesn't have to be expensive. Cod, for example, is generally inexpensive and provides useful amounts of protein and calcium. Eating more fruits and vegetables and less meat will save you money and provide important vitamins and minerals. Because fruits and vegetables lose most of their nutrients when processed you need to buy them fresh or quick frozen, or grow your own. Many shops will home deliver if transport and mobility is a problem.

LIFESTYLE

PROBLEM 1
A more sedentary lifestyle

Many people underestimate the number of calories burnt simply by going to work each day and find they gain weight with inactivity.

SOLUTION

Plan your retirement around staying physically and mentally active. Take up a hobby such as gardening or a sport like golf, bowls or swimming, but also consider other activities to keep you mobile and active. Joining a voluntary organisation or charity, for example, can help focus your day, get you out of the house and help prevent the boredom which can lead to snacking. Use your extra free time to walk more often: to the local shops or to visit friends.

PROBLEM 2
Exercise is painful

The onset of arthritis and other age-related illnesses can discourage people from exercise.

SOLUTION

Although exercise may be painful at first, it is particularly beneficial for arthritis sufferers. Doing warm-up stretches before exercising can reduce pain. Ask your doctor for advice on exercise options. A non-weight-bearing activity such as swimming can ease the strain on joints, while a weight-bearing one (such as walking) can help to strengthen bones. Massage can also help to loosen joints before exercise and ease any pain afterwards.

Weight can be a problem for many retired people, who have to overcome a number of potential threats to their waistlines. Not only does metabolism slow down with age, making the body slower at burning energy, but retirement can also lead to inactivity, while arthritis and other age-related illnesses can make exercise difficult. A reduced income may mean you have to compromise on food, but keeping an allotment or vegetable garden can provide both fresh vegetables and regular exercise. Many older people find themselves eating alone and don't make as much effort to cook fresh food. With careful planning, however, retirement does not always have to lead to weight gain.

YOUR EATING HABITS

Changing your eating patterns takes determination and willpower. First you need to assess honestly what you currently eat and find ways to improve your habits at work and at home.

In order to make a permanent change in your eating habits you need to assess the content of your current diet, and when you are in the habit of eating your meals. Armed with this information, you can decide whether these food habits are conducive to reaching and maintaining your ideal weight.

WHAT YOU REALLY EAT

As discussed in Chapter 4, effective weight control is largely about controlling the level of fat in your diet. However, many people remain ignorant about how much fat they actually eat. It is easy to convince yourself that your current diet is reasonably healthy unless you take the time to list everything you eat and examine the fat content. Keep a food diary for a week (see page 47), noting exactly what you ate, when you ate it, and how much exercise you did during the week. Use the food charts on page 66 and the fat formula on page 73, to work out what percentage of your diet is fat and aim to keep it at around 30 per cent of your total daily intake. Take more time to read food labels and familiarise yourself with products which are truly low in fat; soon you will find buying healthy food items becomes natural.

RECOGNISING YOUR DANGER TIMES

Snacking excessively between meals is the downfall of many people, even when they are eating carefully planned main meals. In order to break the habit, you need to understand the reasons behind it. Common causes include boredom and depression and you should be able to take steps to control your impulses by identifying the periods when you are most likely to reach for a high-fat snack.

If you can see a pattern of snacking during stressful periods at work, for example, force yourself to take a break rather than reaching for a snack. Take the time to perform a few easy stretches or make a cup of tea. Even a brisk walk up and down stairs, around the office or along the road, can break your stress/food cycle.

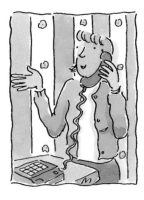

CHEER YOURSELF UP
There is often a link between snacking and being lonely, bored or depressed. Rather than reaching for comfort food, find an activity, such as phoning or writing to a friend, that will lift your mood.

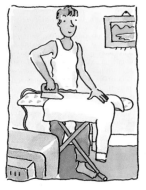

KEEP BUSY
If your danger period is at night while watching television, try to do something more active during this time. If there is a programme you want to see, do something useful, such as ironing, while you watch TV to keep you busy and prevent snacking.

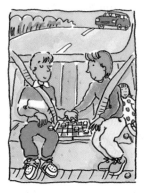

ALLEVIATE BOREDOM
Children often get bored during long journeys, but don't placate them with sweets. Take some travel games instead, or play memory games and catch up on their news of school. Take some fruit so that you are prepared if they get hungry.

A Young Family

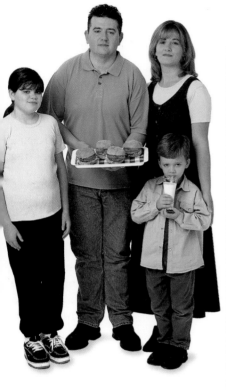

I f you have a family you will find it difficult to initiate new eating habits for yourself without changing your family's habits at the same time. The least successful diets are those that require you to eat in isolation from your family, cooking one meal for them, and another for yourself. Because low-fat foods are not just better for your weight but also contribute to good health, changing dietary habits is important for the whole family. You should aim to change your family's preference for high-sugar and high-fat foods and get their support for your long-term goal.

FOOD

PROBLEM 1
Nutrition needs for children
Your new low-fat diet may create unforeseen nutritional problems for your children.

SOLUTION
Because children are still growing, they should not have their calorie intake restricted, but it is important to introduce them to healthy eating habits as well as ensuring that you are not alienated at mealtimes. Ensure they are getting the necessary calcium for growth by adapting your own meals for them. Keep a supply of full-fat milk for the children and half-fat milk for yourself. Add cheese to your low-fat salads, or if you are serving jacket potatoes, make fillings more calcium-rich for the children using creamy sauces and tuna, while you fill your potato with just tuna and sweetcorn.

PROBLEM 2
Finicky eating
Your children, and even your partner, may resist or oppose changes to their favourite meals.

SOLUTION
Adjusting your family's favourite recipes, reducing fat where possible, is a clever way of subtly changing habits. Gradually cut down the amount of sugar in desserts, and check the amount of sugar in other items you buy. Try to make favourites such as burgers healthier by using a vegetarian burger mix, wholemeal bread and lots of salad.

LIFESTYLE

PROBLEM 1
Lazy family habits
The family as a whole may prefer relaxing and watching television to being active.

SOLUTION
Gradually wean your family away from the television. Begin by playing board games, then move on to more active pursuits that are also fun such as swimming or even rollerblading.

PROBLEM 2
Your partner doesn't support your plan
If your partner is overweight, he or she may have a vested interest in keeping you plump. A partner may even 'sabotage' your best efforts by bringing home treats of chocolate or cakes, or takeaways to 'relieve' you of the burden of cooking.

SOLUTION
Discuss your goals with your partner. Make sure he or she understands the importance of what you are trying to do, and some of the principles of healthy, low-fat eating and exercise that you are trying to introduce. Try to involve your partner in menu planning and exercise ideas. Perhaps he or she has a favourite sport you could share in.

If your partner brings home treats try to maintain your self control. Explain to your partner that these treats make your task harder, and that while the occasional treat is fine, if this happens on a regular basis it will undermine your eating plan.

Low-fat cooking

Use low-fat spreads instead of butter or margarine wherever possible. Egg yolks are high in cholesterol so limit your intake of eggs to two or three a week, and boil, poach or scramble them rather than serving them fried. Choose tuna canned in water rather than oil. Substitute low-fat crème fraîche or yoghurt for butter on jacket potatoes and for cream to accompany fruit. Choose sorbet or low-fat frozen yoghurt for dessert rather than ice cream. If you can't remove cakes and biscuits from your diet completely, try to cut back on cakes with icing or cream, and look at ones that gain their moisture from fruit, rather than butter or eggs. Think about the way you cook and prepare foods as well. For example, grate cheese for sandwiches rather than cutting slices; you will use less cheese. Try to avoid frying food, but if you do, use a non-stick pan, as little oil as possible and lay the cooked food on absorbent paper to remove any excess fat.

MEAL PLANNING

Most successful dieters report that a major part of their success was due to eating regular meals, and carefully considering content to maximise necessary nutrients and taste, while minimising unnecessary fat. Everything you eat contains calories; if you are restricting your calorific intake you need to be especially careful to ensure that you are getting the right balance of nutrients. If your existing diet is high in fat, you may have to plan every meal, checking fat and calories to ensure a proper balance until low-fat

Pathway to health

As you become involved in eating a healthier diet you may enjoy trying new recipes and exploring the cuisines of different cultures. Contact your local education authority for a list of evening courses in your district. Vegetarian, Mediterranean, Korean, and Japanese cuisines can all be low in fat. You may find that attending classes also helps your motivation and lifts your mood, as well as providing a new skill with which to entertain your friends.

eating becomes second nature to you. As you start to exert greater control over what you eat be sure to construct your meals around filling, low-fat complex carbohydrates that will diminish your hunger pangs, as well as giving you the right levels of energy. Pasta dishes, crusty wholemeal bread, potatoes and brown rice, are all useful foods for helping you feel satisfied, and keeping your body well fuelled.

INTRODUCING CHANGES

For many people the stumbling block to changing eating habits is taste. If you have grown up eating predominantly fatty or sugary foods changing your habits is going to mean changing your food preferences. The best way to do this is gradually, giving your body time to adjust to a slow reduction in sugar and fat, rather than immediately cutting out all your favourite types of food. If a favourite meal is high in fat, first try to reduce the frequency with which you have the meal. If you regularly have a 'take away' treat, think about how you could cook the same meal at home – burgers, fish and chips, pizzas and kebabs can all be made at home with healthier, lower calorie ingredients. Next, try to cut down on the amount you eat; portion sizes of take-away food are often much larger than you would eat at home. Many people have a sweet tooth so when it comes to cutting back on sugar it can be difficult to make changes like replacing ice-cream with yoghurt. Start off by serving fresh fruit with your ice-cream. Then serve fresh fruit with flavoured yoghurt, gradually changing to low-fat, natural yoghurt as you develop a taste for less sugar.

HEALTHY FISH AND CHIPS

You don't have to ban your favourite food from passing your lips, but you should look at ways of adapting it to reduce its calories and fat content. These 'fish and chips' are cooked at home – the fish is grilled and the potatoes are sliced and baked (alternatively you could use low-fat oven chips).

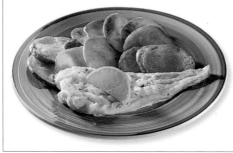

A HEALTHY MEAL Grilled cod can be delicious on its own, without a high-fat batter coating. Use pepper, paprika or lemon juice to give it an extra tang.

An Office Worker

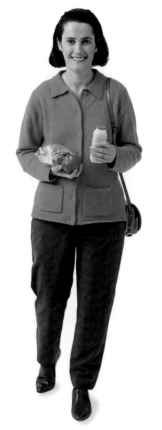

A lthough many people spend most of their lives in an office, few realise how much the office environment can influence eating and exercise patterns. Most office jobs involve being seated for most of the day and provide few opportunities for more activity. At the same time it may be hard to resist high-fat temptations from the staff canteen or neaby cafés. Your will-power can also be sorely tested by the snacking habits of co-workers, expense lunches at restaurants or social occasions after work.

FOOD

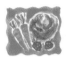

PROBLEM 1
High-fat lunches
You may face temptations of high-calorie foods at the staff canteen or from sandwich bars and cafés nearby.

SOLUTION
Take time to study the menu at the canteen or sandwich bar and work out the options that are lowest in fat. Look at sandwich and salad options rather than quiche or pies which will be high in fat because of their pastry content. Try to prepare your own lunch two or three times a week (see page 128). That way you can control the nutritional content and will probably also save money. Choose high-fibre bread and high-protein, low-fat fillings such as tuna or skinless chicken. Try to keep butter and dressings to a minimum.

PROBLEM 2
Snacking during the day
It's easy to give yourself treats or energy boosts during the day that quickly add calories.

SOLUTION
Look at low-fat beverages, such as herbal tea or mineral water, as an alternative to food. If you must have a snack, try to replace biscuits and cakes with fruit or rice cakes. The natural sweetness of fruit will satisfy your craving for sweet foods, and the saving in calories and fat is significant. Replacing your morning slice of coffee cake with two fresh plums will save over 150 calories and 5 g of fat.

LIFESTYLE

PROBLEM 1
Lack of activity
If your job is desk-based you may be forced to sit for extended periods throughout the day leading to a slowing down of your metabolism. Your job may also provide few 'natural' opportunities for exercise.

SOLUTION
Use the time you do have during the day for exercise. Try to set aside part of your lunchtime for some form of exercise. Organising work colleagues to join you one day a week at a nearby gym can help provide motivation to maintain the exercise. On the other days of the week, try to do a 20 minute brisk walk at lunchtime. You could also try to set up an after work sports match such as football or softball.

PROBLEM 2
Boredom
If you work at your desk for most of the day, and have a predictable work routine, you may become bored and use food as a diversion.

SOLUTION
You should take regular breaks from sitting at your desk to stretch your muscles (see page 30), and re-focus your eyes away from the computer screen. In many offices this is now a health and safety requirement. Try discussing with your manager ways to increase your responsibility or vary your duties. This should help to relieve boredom and avoid your need for snacks.

Packed Lunches

Much of the success of a weight-control plan rests on planning and controlling your food. By taking your own lunch to work, you can control your calorie intake, whereas visiting local eateries can tempt you into eating high-fat foods.

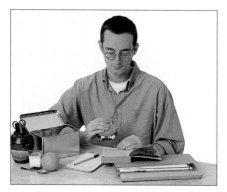

TAKING TIME OUT
Take a break from work at lunchtime to enjoy the food you have prepared.

Sandwiches are the obvious choice for a light, nutritious lunch at work. When making your own, try to limit your fat intake. Avoid butter and margarine altogether, or substitute a low-fat spread and spread it thinly or on one slice of bread only.

Breads are an important source of fibre, protein, iron and calcium – but they vary in fat and calorie content. Wholemeal bread is the healthiest choice, packed with fibre, while breads like foccacia with a high oil content should be avoided.

THE CALORIE AND FAT CONTENT OF BREAD PER 100 g

Pumpernickel = 221 calories, 0.9 g fat

Baguette = 258 calories, 1.5 g fat

Rye = 219 calories, 1.7 g fat

White bagel = 275 calories, 1.5 g fat

White pitta = 265 calories, 1.2 g fat

Wholemeal pitta = 223 calories, 1.7 g fat

Brown soda = 258 calories, 2.5 g fat

Granary loaf = 235 calories, 2.7 g fat

LOW-FAT SANDWICH FILLINGS

When selecting your sandwich fillers, consider the consistency of the bread to avoid a soggy and unappetising lunch. Unless the bread is crusty, 'wet' vegetables such as tomatoes and cucumber will soak into bread, and the sandwich will collapse. Try the following combinations:

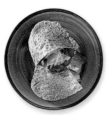

Grated cheese, grated carrot and spinach leaves on pitta bread = about 373 calories

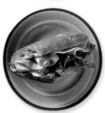

Lean honey-cured ham, lettuce and sun-dried tomato paste on a baguette = about 171 calories

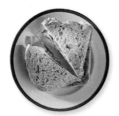

Smoked turkey, rocket leaves and mango chutney on granary bread = about 170 calories

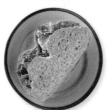

Sardines, long green beans and raddichio on soda bread = about 277 calories

SALAD LUNCHES

Salad lunches make an ideal alternative to sandwiches. Buy a crusty wholegrain bun, some low-fat cheese, cherry tomatoes, shredded salad greens, and add leftovers from meals. For example, if you are cooking beans or broccoli for the evening meal, cook some extra for your salad for the next day.

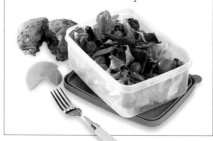

Self-Assessment

Once your weight-control plan is successfully underway, it is important to monitor your progress so that you can see how well the programme is working.

You should monitor the rate at which you are losing weight, aiming for a gradual loss: a weight loss of 0.5 to 1 kg (about 1 to 2 lb) a week is a sensible goal. If you lose in excess of 2 kg (4.5 lb) a week you are losing weight too fast and should moderate your programme, or risk compromising your health. It is also important that you recognise when you should stop trying to lose weight and concentrate on weight maintenance instead.

GAUGING YOUR SUCCESS

For most people the scales are the ultimate arbiter of whether their weight-control plan has been successful or not. But scales can be a source of tyranny. While it is useful to check progress in this way, be reasonable in your expectations. Don't weigh yourself more than once a week and bear in mind that early rapid weight loss, while encouraging, is likely to be simple fluid loss. Sustained weight loss, when stored supplies of fat begin to be used by the body, will take longer to occur.

Weight alone is not the only guide to your progress in your new healthy lifestyle. If you have introduced a fitness programme you should measure your increased levels of fitness as well. An improved resting heart rate and improved recovery rate (see page 79) from exercise are measurable, and will show you that you are making progress in raising your metabolic rate and therefore helping to burn fat faster.

Even when the scales show that your weight is not falling, you may in fact have shed fat but have added muscle bulk. You can test whether your shape has changed by trying on tight-fitting skirts or trousers and seeing whether they have loosened a little or hang any better.

On the other hand, be wary of gauging success in the mirror. You are not the most objective assessor of your own appearance. Evidence suggests that people distort the image they actually see in the mirror. Even someone in the healthy weight range for their age and height can perceive their mirror image to be overweight.

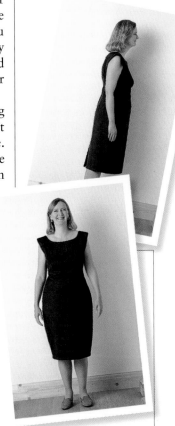

TELL-TALE ANGLES
Your shape looks different from the front and profile so take one photo facing the camera and one side-on.

SETTING UP A SENSIBLE 'BEFORE' SNAPSHOT

Weighing yourself is not the only way to judge the success of your weight-control programme. For most people, looking slim and fitting easily into their clothes is the main motivation for dieting. A picture of you at the beginning of your plan will help boost your morale in the months ahead when you see how much you have achieved. Here are some tips on setting up a realistic 'before' photo:

▶ *If your camera has a self-timer mechanism, you can take the pictures yourself: set the camera up on a tripod or on a table top. Check the position by marking your height*

on the wall, or using something the same height as yourself as a stand-in. Alternatively, ask a friend to take the picture for you.

▶ *Find an uncluttered background against which to take the photo so that there are no distractions from your figure. A blank wall is ideal – stand about a foot away from it.*

▶ *Wear close-fitting, plain-coloured clothes. Large patterns such as stripes and spots can cause optical illusions making you appear bigger than you really are.*

▶ *Use a flash if possible. Otherwise, stand close to a window, so there is plenty of light, or take the picture outdoors.*

DANGER SIGNS OF EATING DISORDERS

Obsessive dieting can lead to eating disorders such as anorexia and bulimia. If you experience any of the danger signals listed below, consult your doctor immediately.

▶ *Missing three consecutive menstrual periods.*

▶ *Self-induced vomiting.*

▶ *Binge eating, especially of junk food, accompanied by mood swings.*

▶ *Food hoarding.*

▶ *Eating in secret.*

▶ *Depression and loss of sleep.*

▶ *Significant weight fluctuations – 4.5 kg (10 lb) or more over a month.*

▶ *Dramatic weight loss over a short period of time.*

Unfortunately, this can be taken to extremes – research conducted with anorexia nervosa sufferers has shown that they consistently see themselves as fatter than they actually are, to the point where young girls who are emaciated still see themselves as being overweight in the mirror. Rather than simply relying on the subjectivity of the mirror, gauge your success through things that are objectively measurable: weighing yourself, testing your fitness level, and measuring with a tape measure.

As an alternative to the mirror, have a snapshot taken of yourself (see page 129) at the beginning of your weight-control programme. After three months take a photograph wearing the same clothing and using the same lighting. The photographs can provide a more objective measurement of change. A photograph may also show you what part of your body you have a tendency to lose weight from first. Because our body shape determines fat distribution (see page 118), you will probably first lose weight from areas you may not be targeting. For example, a mesomorph woman may lose weight from her face and breasts rather than thighs and buttocks. Don't be disheartened if this is what your snapshot shows you. Be encouraged that you are losing weight, and consider how to revise your exercise programme to firm up problem areas.

Warning signs

If you are following a sensible, healthy eating plan and exercising, your 'diet' should never become dangerous. It is when dieting becomes an obsession that you should step back and assess more objectively your behaviour. If you feel fatigued and lethargic this is a sign that you have an insufficient energy intake for your needs. Ensure you have an adequate intake of complex carbohydrates to function properly. Anorexia and bulimia can develop from obsessive dieting.

Maintaining your new weight

Few people can, or should, maintain the demands of a severely calorie-controlled diet. Long term, permanent weight loss results from a shift in eating habits to low-fat options and the introduction of exercise. Successful dieters are those who can still follow the broad principles of their weight-control plan, without feeling they are being forced to make unsustainable changes to

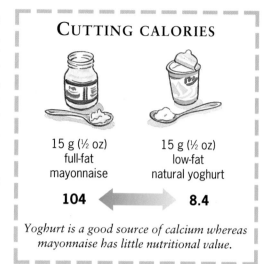

CUTTING CALORIES

15 g (½ oz) full-fat mayonnaise

15 g (½ oz) low-fat natural yoghurt

104 ◀▬▶ **8.4**

Yoghurt is a good source of calcium whereas mayonnaise has little nutritional value.

their lifestyle. Remember that you can't return to your old eating habits. Once you have lost weight your body needs less fuel to function efficiently. A rough rule of thumb is that for every pound of weight lost, you should eat ten fewer calories.

FEELING CONTENT

As your eating habits improve and you start to exercise regularly you should soon feel and see the benefits to your body. Your skin will improve with the increased intake of vitamin C and A from fresh fruit and vegetables, and exercise should improve your sleeping patterns which will in turn help the restorative functions of the body. With an improved oxygen flow from exercise you will experience increased vitality and energy. Regular exercise will also firm and tone your muscles. All these factors should combine to make you look and feel better than you did before you started. Even if you haven't met your target weight, you will have made substantial improvements to your health and well-being. You may have difficulty in shedding the last few kilos to reach your target weight and will need to consider whether an increase in your exercise intensity is worthwhile. On reflection you may find you are content with what you have achieved.

Be wary of over-reacting to criticism from others. Remember, the most important element in your weight-control plan is your own health and happiness. If you have achieved a weight within the BMI range for your height and are following sensible eating and exercise principles, you should be more than satisfied with the result.

CHAPTER 9

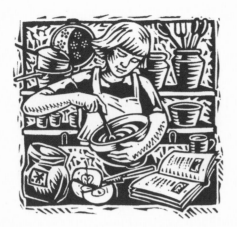

RECIPES
FOR WEIGHT
CONTROL

This chapter offers a selection of delicious low-fat
calorie-controlled recipes that will appeal to both the
weightwatcher and the non-dieter. Many of the dishes
are ideal for entertaining as well as for family meals.
Calorie and fat amounts per serving are given for each
recipe. Check pages 66–67 for calorific values of any
additional accompaniments. Ingredients are given in
both metric and imperial measures, but they are not
precise equivalents, so use either all-metric or
all-imperial measures for any given recipe.

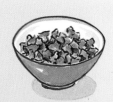

BREAKFASTS

If you are not really a lover of breakfast, it can be tempting to cut out this first meal of the day. The advantages seem many: extra time in bed, a reduction in the total number of calories you eat each day, or being able to eat more at another meal time. However, breakfast really is the most important meal of the day.

Breakfast is exactly what the word implies – breaking a fast. By early morning it is usually many hours since you have eaten anything, causing the sugar level in your blood to be very low. Food is needed to replenish the body's carbohydrate stores – if the level remains low, by mid-morning you can end up feeling faint, lacking in concentration and have a craving for food. This is when you reach for a mid-morning snack, which is all too likely to be high-calorie convenience foods such as biscuits, cakes, chocolate or crisps.

Breakfast is the ideal time to eat foods that are rich in complex carbohydrates to provide your body with energy for the day. The recipes and menu ideas that follow emphasise a high content of fibre, protein and carbohydrate with plenty of vital micronutrients.

All the family can sit down to the same breakfast, but those who are not watching their weight can eat a combination of more items and not necessarily low-calorie varieties. This may involve buying a variety of cereals and low-fat spread as well as butter. Children under five should always be given full-fat milk to drink and to have with cereal, while skimmed or semi-skimmed milk can be used by the rest of the family to reduce their fat intake.

COMPLETE BREAKFAST IDEAS

If your breakfast provides enough energy it should see you through until lunchtime. Each of the following breakfast menu suggestions provides a filling meal to start the day that is not too high in calories.

MENU 1

Half a grapefruit provides more than half of an adult's daily requirement for vitamin C.

½ grapefruit
raisin porridge (see recipe, right)
tea/coffee (with skimmed milk or a slice of lemon)

210 cals, 3 g fat

MENU 2

Eggs are rich in protein, vitamins and minerals but are high in cholesterol so try not to choose eggs every day.

250 ml/9 fl oz orange juice
25 g/1 oz wholewheat muesli with
semi-skimmed milk
1 egg, scrambled, served with 1 slice of rye bread, toasted

398 cals, 15 g fat

MENU 3

If you prefer a cooked breakfast, fish will provide a rich source of low-fat protein to set you up for the day.

115 g/4 oz white fish such as haddock, served with
1 tomato (grilled)
1 slice of wholemeal bread
tea/coffee (with skimmed milk or a slice of lemon)

208 cals, 2.5 g fat

MENU 4

Yoghurt is an excellent source of calcium and strawberries provide a useful source of vitamin C.

muesli (see recipe, right)
225 g/8 oz low-fat yoghurt with 3 strawberries (sliced)
tea/coffee (with skimmed milk or a slice of lemon)

443 cals, 12 g fat

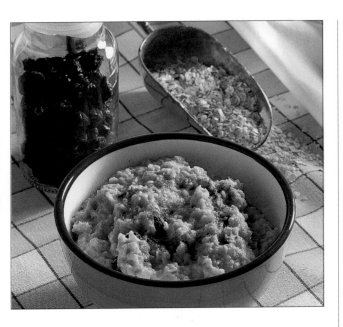

OAT, FRUIT AND NUT MUESLI

304 cals, 10 g fat per serving
Serves 4

The fruits, nuts and seeds in this recipe provide a range of nutrients while the sugar in the dried fruit lends natural sweetness.

115 g/4 oz mixed dried fruits such as raisins, sultanas, ready-to-eat apricots and prunes
55 g/2 oz mixed nuts and seeds such as walnuts and sunflower seeds
115 g/4 oz porridge oats
2 pieces of fresh fruit such as an apple, orange or soft fruit in season

■ Cut up any large pieces of dried fruit and nuts and mix all the ingredients except the fresh fruit together in a large mixing bowl. You can store some of the mixture in an air-tight container if you do not need it all.
■ To serve, prepare the fresh fruit as appropriate, add a quarter of the muesli mix and pour over semi-skimmed milk or low-fat yoghurt.

RAISIN PORRIDGE

177 cals, 2.5 g fat per serving
Serves 4

Porridge can always be relied upon to provide a warming start to the day and is an excellent source of soluble fibre.

300 ml/10 fl oz skimmed milk
600 ml/1 pint water
55 g/2 oz seedless raisins
large pinch cinnamon
115 g/4 oz quick porridge oats

■ Place the milk, water, raisins and cinnamon in a saucepan and bring to the boil. Stir in the oats then reduce the heat and simmer for about 5 minutes until the mixture thickens, stirring occasionally to prevent it sticking to the pan.

DAILY MEAL PLAN

BREAKFAST: *Menu 1 (page 132)*
MID-MORNING SNACK: *Banana*
LUNCH: *Crunchy Salad with Vinaigrette (page 139) with 1 slice of wholemeal pitta bread; mineral water*
DINNER: *Stuffed Aubergines (page 147) with 55 g/2 oz broccoli, 100 g/3½ oz carrots and 150 g/5½ oz boiled new potatoes; 350 ml/12 fl oz fresh fruit juice*
DESSERT: *Coeur à la Crème (page 156); herbal tea*

TOTAL FOR THE DAY: 1406 calories, 31.5 g fat

As the total calories for the day are low you could have a glass of wine or 300 ml/10 fl oz of beer with your dinner. This would add about 95 calories to the total.

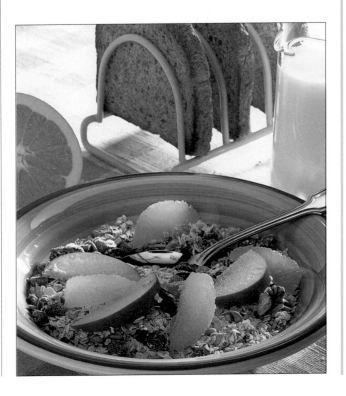

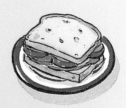

LIGHT MEALS AND SNACKS

When watching your weight it is often difficult to think of what to eat for a light meal or snack. It is all too easy to reach for convenience foods like biscuits, crisps and takeaways – which are high in both fat and calories and can ruin your weight control plan.

Try some of the recipes on the following pages for a low-fat calorie controlled choice. Several of the light meals can be turned into main meals if desired. The salads can form a light meal in their own right, or be eaten with low-fat cheese or cold meat. Additionally, they can be served as accompaniments to one of the main meals given on pages 142–149. The Chinese Stir-Fried Vegetables on page 137 can also be enjoyed with a main course if calories allow. Salad dressings often add an unhealthy amount of fat to an otherwise healthy eating choice. Try the vinaigrette that accompanies the crunchy salad on page 139, or concoct a low-fat dressing of your own: yoghurt and fromage frais make good bases for dressings, thinned with a little water and flavoured with fresh herbs and a flavoured vinegar such as raspberry, tarragon or sherry vinegar. When you do use an oil to make a dressing, avoid oils that are high in saturates: olive oil, hazelnut oil and walnut oil are all good choices, but remember that all oils contain the same amount of calories.

If you don't have time to prepare one of these recipes, sandwiches are a practical healthy alternative. Be careful when buying ready-made sandwiches as the fillings used can often be high in fat – avoid bacon, avocado, full-fat cheese, and fillings such as coleslaw that use mayonnaise as a binding ingredient. If possible, make your own sandwiches (see page 128) and increase the ratio of bread to filling by slicing your bread thicker.

TIGER PRAWN FAJITAS WITH SALSA

456 cals, 3 g fat per serving
Serves 4

Prawns are a good low-fat source of protein. Here, soured cream and guacamole have been replaced by coriander salsa and yoghurt, which are low in fat.

450 g/1 lb raw tiger prawns, peeled, deveined and defrosted
zest and juice of 1 lime
1 clove garlic, crushed
½ red chilli, deseeded and very finely chopped
1 tbsp freshly chopped coriander
salt and freshly ground black pepper
1 bunch spring onions
12 soft flour tortillas
1 red and 1 yellow pepper, quartered and deseeded
150 g/5½ oz low-fat natural yoghurt or smatana

For the coriander salsa
3 tbsp freshly chopped coriander
½ red chilli, deseeded and very finely chopped
zest and juice of 1 lime

■ Preheat the oven to 180°C/350°F/Gas mark 4. Place the prawns in a bowl with the lime zest and juice, garlic, chilli, coriander and seasoning, and leave to marinate.
■ For the salsa: finely chop two spring onions and mix with the coriander, chilli, lime zest and juice. Season and set aside.
■ Wrap the tortillas in foil and warm in the oven for 15 minutes.
■ Grill the peppers until the skins begin to char. Leave to cool slightly, remove the skins and slice into strips. Cut the rest of the onions into slivers and arrange on a platter with the peppers.
■ Heat a large non-stick frying pan over a high heat. Remove the prawns from the marinade and put them into the frying pan. Stir-fry until they turn pink and are cooked through.
■ Spread some smatana on a warm tortilla, add a few prawns, top with the spring onions, peppers and salsa and roll up.

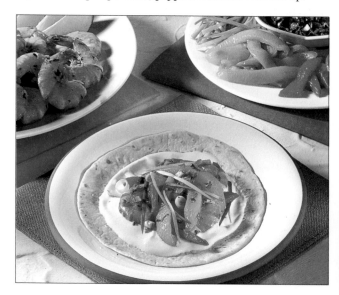

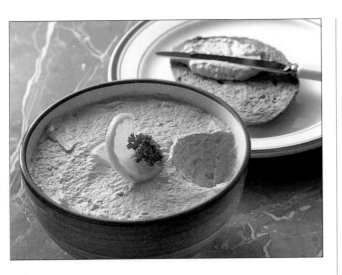

SMOKED MACKEREL PÂTÉ

332 cals, 22 g fat per serving
Serves 4

Oily fish is an important component of a balanced diet supplying valuable protein, calcium, vitamin D and omega-3 fatty acids, all essential for good health.

275 g/9½ oz smoked mackerel fillets
115 g/4 oz low-fat cream cheese
150 g/5½ oz low-fat natural yoghurt
juice of half a lemon
2 tsp creamed horseradish
freshly ground black pepper
4 slices of lemon and sprigs of parsley for garnish
4 slices of wholemeal toast to serve

■ Carefully remove any bones from the mackerel, peel off the skin, then break the fish into small pieces.
■ Put all the ingredients together in a blender and combine until the mixture is thick and creamy. Press into a suitable container, such as a bowl from which guests can help themselves, or into four small individual pots.
■ Chill until ready to serve. Garnish with lemon slices and sprigs of parsley and serve with slices of toast.

DAILY MEAL PLAN

BREAKFAST: Menu 3 (page 132)
MID-MORNING SNACK: Wholemeal bread roll with 55 g/2 oz cottage cheese
LUNCH: Smoked Mackerel Pâté with toast; 330 ml/ 11 fl oz fresh orange juice
DINNER: Chinese Chicken (page 148) with 150 g/5½ oz boiled rice; glass of mineral water
DESSERT: Melon Surprise (page 153); cup of herbal tea

TOTAL FOR THE DAY: 1297 calories, 33.5 g fat

MEDITERRANEAN TOMATO SOUP

111 cals, 6.5 g fat per serving
Serves 4

Soup makes a filling meal and is very nutritious because the cooking process does not rob the vegetables of their vitamins. This low-calorie soup is rich in potassium, beta-carotene and vitamin E.

900 g/2 lb plum tomatoes
2 tbsp olive oil
1 small onion, skinned and chopped
½ large red pepper, deseeded and chopped
1 clove garlic, crushed
2 tbsp red wine
2 tsp freshly chopped basil plus 4 sprigs for garnish
300 ml/10 fl oz hot chicken or vegetable stock
salt and freshly ground black pepper

■ Place the tomatoes in a bowl, pour boiling water over them and leave them for a few moments. Remove from the boiling water with a slotted spoon and cool in a bowl of cold water for a few minutes. Peel off the skins and discard. On a chopping board, quarter the tomatoes and remove and discard the seeds.
■ Heat the oil in a large saucepan and lightly sauté the onion, pepper and garlic. Add the tomatoes, red wine and chopped basil. Bring this mixture to the boil and simmer gently for about 15 minutes.
■ Transfer the mixture to a liquidiser and blend at top speed until the contents are very smooth. Return the soup to the pan and add the hot stock to thin it to the desired consistency. Season to taste. Divide the soup equally between four serving bowls and serve piping hot garnished with a sprig of basil.

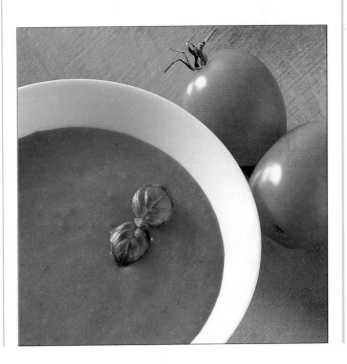

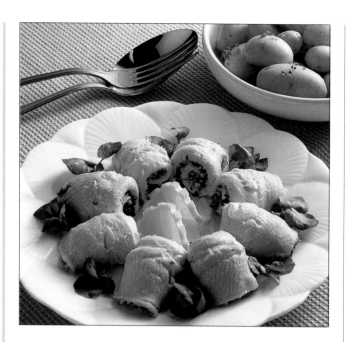

TROUT ROULADES WITH WATERCRESS AND MUSHROOM STUFFING

252 cals, 8.5 g fat per serving

Serves 4

This tasty, filling meal has an incredibly low calorie intake and yet its nutritional value is high, providing potassium and vitamins A, C and D.

15 g/½ oz low-fat margarine
4 spring onions, finely chopped
75 g/2¾ oz watercress, chopped
75 g/2¾ oz mushrooms, finely chopped
75 g/2¾ oz wholemeal breadcrumbs
2 tbsp lemon juice
salt and freshly ground black pepper
4 trout fillets each weighing about 150 g/5½ oz
4 lemon wedges and sprigs of parsley for garnish

■ Preheat the oven to 190°C/375°F/Gas mark 5. Heat the margarine in a non-stick frying pan until melted. Add the onion, watercress and mushrooms and fry gently for about 5 minutes. Stir in the breadcrumbs and half the lemon juice and mix together well. Season to taste then leave to one side while you prepare the fish.
■ Skin the fillets and lay them flat on a board with the skinned side uppermost. Cut each fillet in half lengthwise and sprinkle them with the remaining lemon juice. Divide the stuffing into eight, placing it along the centre of each fillet. Roll up from the tail end and secure firmly with a cocktail stick. Place a large piece of foil on a baking tray. Lightly grease the foil, place the fillets on top, then fold the foil over to seal as a parcel.
■ Bake in the oven for 20–25 minutes, or until the fish is cooked through, and then remove the cocktail sticks. Arrange the stuffed fillets on a serving dish and garnish with the lemon wedges and parsley.

FARFALLE WITH BROCCOLI AND FRESH TOMATOES

369 cals, 4 g fat per serving

Serves 2

This quick dish can be put together in the time it takes to boil the pasta, and the fresh ingredients are full of vitamins and flavour. Broccoli is a particularly good source of folic acid, vitamin C and beta-carotene.

175 g/6 oz white farfalle or other dried pasta shapes
175 g/6 oz ripe plum tomatoes
1 tsp olive oil
1 red chilli, deseeded and finely chopped
1 clove garlic, crushed
175 g/6 oz broccoli, separated into florets
2 tbsp freshly chopped basil
salt and freshly ground black pepper

■ Put the pasta on to boil in plenty of boiling salted water.
■ Place the tomatoes in a bowl, pour boiling water over them and leave them for a few moments. Remove from the boiling water with a slotted spoon and cool in a bowl of cold water for a few minutes. Peel off the skins and discard. On a chopping board, quarter the tomatoes, remove and discard the seeds, and chop roughly.
■ In a small pan, gently infuse the oil with the chilli and garlic over a low heat, without browning.
■ Blanch the broccoli florets in boiling salted water for 3 minutes, then drain.
■ Turn up the heat under the chilli and garlic oil, add the basil, tomatoes and plenty of seasoning, and cook for 1 minute.
■ Drain the cooked pasta and mix it together with the broccoli and tomato mixture and serve in deep bowls. For a main meal, increase the quantity of pasta to 225 g/8 oz and serve with a fresh green salad.

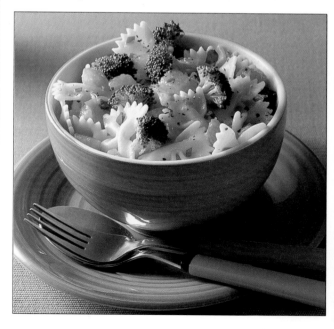

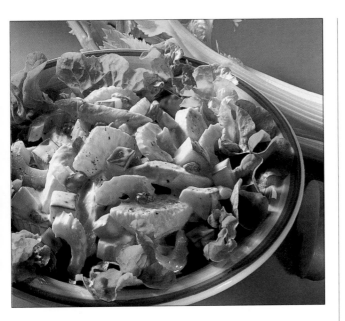

CHICKEN AND CELERY SALAD

287 cals, 6.5 g fat per serving

Serves 4

Lean chicken is an excellent source of protein, vitamins and minerals. Here, it is combined with a mixture of fruit and vegetables for extra nutritional value.

450 g/1 lb cooked chicken
8 sticks celery, cut into bite-size pieces
2 red eating apples
2 tbsp lemon juice
55 g/2 oz sultanas
1 large grapefruit, peeled and segmented
300 g/10½ oz low-fat natural yoghurt
salt and freshly ground black pepper
1 small head of lettuce, split into leaves

■ Remove and discard any skin from the chicken and cut into thick strips; add to a bowl with the celery. Core and dice the apples, place them in another small bowl and sprinkle with the lemon juice to prevent them from discolouring.
■ Add the sultanas and grapefruit segments to the chicken and celery, followed by the apple and lemon juice. Stir all the ingredients together well. Add the yoghurt and stir well into the mixture. Season to taste with salt and pepper.
■ Arrange the lettuce leaves on a serving dish, pile the chicken mixture on top and refrigerate until ready to serve.

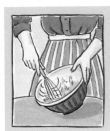

HEALTHY EATING TIP
Most of the fat content of chicken comes from the skin so always use skinless chicken and use breast meat where possible as it is lower in fat than chicken wings or drumsticks.

CHINESE STIR-FRIED VEGETABLES

188.5 cals, 11.5 g fat per serving

Serves 4

Whatever your diet restrictions, fresh vegetables can always be eaten in unlimited amounts adding essential vitamins, minerals and dietary fibre to the diet.

55 g/2 oz whole almonds
115 g/4 oz cauliflower, broken into florets
1 tbsp sunflower oil
2 sticks celery, thinly sliced
4 spring onions, thinly sliced
1 medium red pepper, deseeded and cut into thin strips
115 g/4 oz button mushrooms, sliced
115 g/4 oz mangetout peas, topped and tailed
1 tsp fresh ginger, grated, or ½ tsp dried ginger
2 cloves garlic, crushed
300 ml/10 fl oz vegetable stock
1 tsp sesame oil
2 tbsp soy sauce
2 tsp dry sherry (optional)
2 tsp arrowroot
115 g/4 oz bean shoots
coriander sprigs for garnish

■ Dry-fry the almonds or toast them under the grill. Blanch the cauliflower by dropping it into boiling water, boil for 1 minute then drain. Heat the oil in a wok or large frying pan and add the celery, spring onions, red pepper, mushrooms, mangetout, ginger and garlic, stirring and tossing the vegetables until they are just becoming tender.
■ Add the stock, sesame oil, soy sauce and sherry. Continue to toss the ingredients together until the liquid boils. In a cup blend the arrowroot with 1 tbsp of cold water. Add this to the wok and stir until the mixture thickens. Add the cauliflower, bean shoots and almonds. Heat thoroughly and serve immediately, garnished with coriander sprigs.

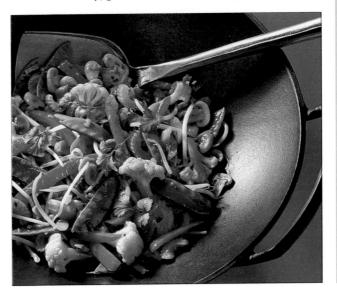

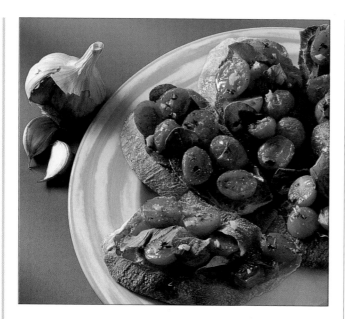

BRUSCHETTA WITH GRILLED TOMATOES AND ROCKET

231 cals, 3 g fat per serving
Serves 2

The Mediterranean diet is recognised as being healthy as well as flavoursome. The freshness of the ingredients is always important – here, grilling the tomatoes brings out their natural sweetness.

225 g/8 oz ripe cherry tomatoes, halved
salt and freshly ground black pepper
2 cloves garlic
2 tsp freshly chopped thyme
4 slices ciabatta bread
25 g/1 oz rocket leaves

■ Place the halved tomatoes on a non-stick baking sheet and season with salt and freshly ground black pepper.
■ Finely chop one garlic clove and scatter over the tomatoes with the thyme. Place under a preheated moderate grill and cook for 5 minutes until the tomatoes have softened and are slightly charred around the edges.
■ Cut the remaining garlic clove in half lengthways. Toast the ciabatta slices and then rub them with the cut sides of garlic. Pile on the rocket leaves and cooked tomatoes and serve immediately.

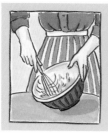

HEALTHY EATING TIP
Although ciabatta is higher in calories than traditional bread, it is a healthy choice as it is made with olive oil which is high in monounsaturated fatty acids that don't raise cholesterol levels.

SAFFRON COUSCOUS SALAD WITH SMOKED TROUT

226 cals, 3 g fat per serving
Serves 4

This salad is colourful and easy to make. It is high in protein and low in fat, using yoghurt as a healthy alternative to an oil-based dressing.

225 g/8 oz couscous
1 tsp ground cumin
½ tsp ground coriander
salt and freshly ground black pepper
3 good pinches saffron
425 ml/15 fl oz vegetable stock
juice of 1 lemon
3 tbsp freshly chopped flat-leaf parsley
½ cucumber, diced
225 g/8 oz cherry tomatoes, quartered
1 small bulb fennel, trimmed and diced
115 g/4 oz carrots, peeled and diced
4 spring onions, finely sliced
2 smoked trout fillets (approximately 150 g/5½ oz total)
3 tbsp low-fat natural yoghurt
3 tbsp freshly chopped mint
pinch of cayenne pepper

■ Put the couscous in a large bowl and stir in the cumin, coriander and some seasoning. Add the saffron to the stock and bring to a boil over medium heat; stir in the lemon juice then pour the hot stock over the couscous and mix well. Leave until the liquid has been absorbed, about 10–15 minutes.
■ Fluff and loosen the couscous with a fork. Mix in the parsley and check for seasoning. Tip into a glass salad bowl.
■ Scatter the vegetables over the couscous and flake the trout fillets over the top.
■ To make the dressing, mix together the yoghurt and mint with a pinch of cayenne and some salt, and serve separately.

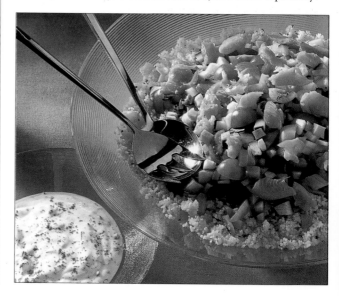

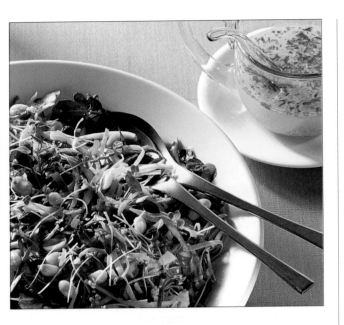

CRUNCHY SALAD WITH VINAIGRETTE

253 cals, 13 g fat per serving
Serves 4

Raw cabbage forms the crunchy base of this salad. It contains more micronutrients than lettuce, is a good source of vitamin C and is high in dietary fibre.

½ small white cabbage
½ small red cabbage
1 bunch watercress
2 medium carrots
1 box mustard-and-cress
4 tbsp raisins
4 tbsp unsalted peanuts
2 tbsp lemon juice

For 225 ml/8 fl oz vinaigrette:
100 ml/3½ fl oz white wine vinegar
100 ml/3½ fl oz lemon juice
1 tbsp olive oil
2 tsp wholegrain mustard
2 tsp honey
1 clove garlic, crushed (optional)
2 tbsp chopped fresh parsley
salt and freshly ground black pepper

■ To make the salad: wash and trim all the vegetables. Finely shred the white and red cabbage, remove the thick stems from the watercress and coarsely grate the carrots. Place all the ingredients in a salad bowl and toss to mix well.
■ To make the vinaigrette: put the vinegar, lemon juice, olive oil, wholegrain mustard, honey, garlic and parsley in a screw-topped jar with a tight-fitting lid and shake to mix well. Add salt and pepper to taste. Serve separately.

BAKED JACKET POTATO

144–242 cals, 1–10 g fat per serving
Serves 1

Baked jacket potatoes are packed with complex carbohydrates and are a great low-fat source of fibre and nutrients.

1 medium potato (about 175g/6 oz)

■ Preheat oven to 220°C/425°F/Gas mark 7. Scrub the potato lightly and dry with a paper towel. Prick in several places with a sharp pointed knife. Bake for 1 hour or until tender.
■ Cut the cooked potato in half lengthways. Scoop out the inside into a basin, taking care not to break the skin. Mix the potato with any of the suggested fillings and season to taste.
■ Pile the mixture back into the potato shell and serve.

FILLINGS

25 g/1 oz mushrooms, chopped and lightly fried
30 calories, 3 g fat per serving

1 scrambled egg and chopped fresh parsley
111 calories, 9.5 g fat per serving

55 g/2 oz chopped cooked spinach and lots of pepper
13 calories, 0.5 g fat per serving

55 g/2 oz flaked canned salmon and sliced tomato
86 calories, 4 g fat per serving

55 g/2 oz canned sardines and cucumber
110 calories, 7 g fat per serving

55 g/2 oz baked beans and 25 g/1 oz grated low-fat Cheddar
107 calories, 4 g fat per serving

25 g/1 oz prawns and watercress
29 calories, 0.5 g fat per serving

25 g/1 oz chopped ham and 1 tbsp sweetcorn
54 calories, 1.5 g fat per serving

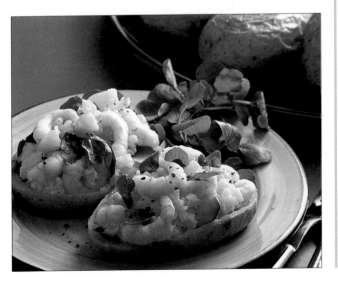

139

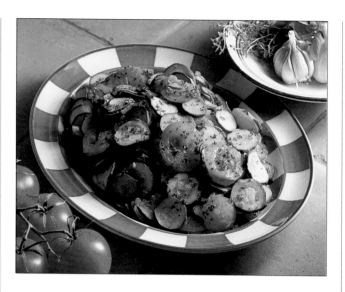

COURGETTES PROVENÇALE

64 cals, 1 g fat per serving
Serves 4

Courgettes are highly nutritious containing good amounts of vitamin C, folate and beta-carotene – most of these nutrients are found in the tender, edible skin.

450 g/1 lb courgettes, thinly sliced
225 g/8 oz onions, skinned and thinly sliced
450 g/1 lb tomatoes, skinned and sliced
1 clove garlic, peeled and crushed
salt and freshly ground black pepper
1 tbsp fresh or dried basil or thyme
2 tbsp chopped parsley for garnish

■ Place all the vegetables, the garlic, the seasoning and basil or thyme into a saucepan, cover and simmer gently until tender, about 15–20 minutes. If the mixture seems to be a bit dry during cooking because the tomatoes were not very juicy, add a little chicken or vegetable stock.
■ Transfer to a warmed serving dish, garnish with the parsley and serve piping hot.

DAILY MEAL PLAN

BREAKFAST: Menu 2 (page 132)
MID-MORNING SNACK: 100 g/3½ oz fresh strawberries with 100 g/3½ oz low-fat natural yoghurt
LUNCH: Courgettes Provençale with 2 slices of wholemeal bread; glass of mineral water
DINNER: Jambalaya (page 149); glass of fruit juice
DESSERT: Baked Stuffed Apples with Home-made Custard (page 155); cup of herbal tea

TOTAL FOR THE DAY: 1487 calories, 33 g fat

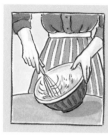

HEALTHY EATING TIP

Eggs are rich in protein, vitamins and minerals. They are best stored in the main part of the refrigerator (instead of the door compartment) where they will keep for about three weeks.

SCRAMBLED EGGS WITH SMOKED SALMON AND COTTAGE CHEESE

361 cals, 15.5 g fat per serving
Serves 1

This is a quick lunch dish with a touch of luxury – delicious slivers of smoked salmon. The scrambled eggs taste extra creamy with the addition of low-fat cottage cheese. For the toast, use a good mixed grain or seeded loaf – the crunchy texture makes all the difference.

2 medium eggs
salt and freshly ground black pepper
2 small slices of mixed grain bread
2 tbsp low-fat cottage cheese
40 g/1½ oz smoked salmon, cut into thin strips
sprigs of fresh chives to garnish

■ Beat the eggs in a small bowl with a little salt and pepper. Heat a non-stick saucepan over a gentle heat and add the eggs. Cook over a gentle heat, stirring continuously.
■ Toast the bread.
■ When the eggs are nearly cooked, stir in the cottage cheese and mix in well. Add the smoked salmon and tip straight on to the toast, before the eggs overcook. Garnish with chives.

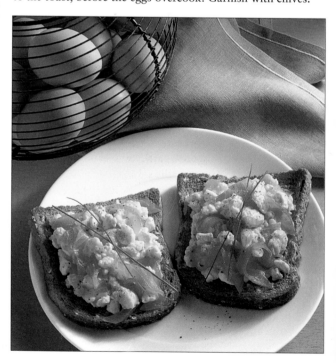

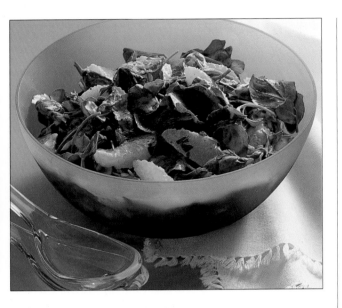

WATERCRESS AND ORANGE SALAD

90 cals, 3.5 g fat per serving
Serves 4

The watercress and oranges provide vitamin C in this colourful and refreshing dish, and the watercress also adds a little iron.

1 bunch watercress
2 large oranges
12 freshly cracked hazelnuts if available or
   2 tbsp chopped hazelnuts
150 g/5½ oz low-fat natural yoghurt
1 clove garlic, crushed
1 tbsp chopped fresh parsley
salt and freshly ground black pepper

■ Remove any very thick stems from the watercress and separate it into sprigs. Rinse thoroughly in a colander. Peel the oranges and cut into segments making sure all the membrane and pith are removed. Do this over a bowl so that all the juice is saved. Cut the segments in half if they are large. Toss the watercress, orange segments and nuts together and place in a serving bowl.
■ In a separate bowl make the dressing: beat together the reserved orange juice, yoghurt, garlic and parsley and add salt and pepper to taste. Pour over the salad and toss well. Leave to stand for about 20 minutes before serving to allow the flavours to blend and develop.

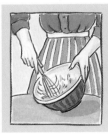

HEALTHY EATING TIP
Both watercress and oranges provide a rich source of vitamin C and beta-carotene. These are antioxidants which can help to protect the body against infections and even cancer.

CHICKEN TIKKA PITTAS WITH A COOL RELISH

447 cals, 8 g per serving
Serves 4

Spicy chicken stuffed into a pitta makes a quick and healthy lunch. Tossing the chicken in yoghurt helps to both tenderise the meat and assist in the absorption of flavours.

4 boneless, skinless chicken breasts, about 150 g/5½ oz each
2 tbsp tikka curry paste
300 g/10½ oz low-fat natural yoghurt
1 cucumber
2 tbsp chopped fresh mint
salt and freshly ground black pepper

To serve:
4 pittas
wedges of lemon

■ Cut each chicken breast into 5 or 6 even-sized chunks. Blend the curry paste with 4 tbsp of the yoghurt and toss the chicken in the mixture until it is well coated. Leave to marinate for at least 15 minutes, or longer if possible.
■ Dice the cucumber into small cubes and toss it with the rest of the yoghurt, the mint and some seasoning. Chill until ready to serve.
■ Preheat the grill and soak 4 wooden skewers in water for 15 minutes to prevent them from burning under the grill.
■ Thread the chicken on to the skewers and season. Cook on a rack under a moderate grill for 10–15 minutes, until the chicken is cooked through and beginning to char at the edges.
■ Meanwhile, warm the pitta breads and split them open. Fill with the yoghurt relish and the chicken tikka. Serve with lemon wedges to squeeze over the chicken.

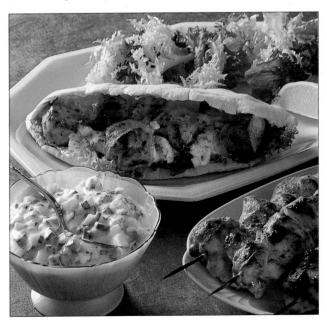

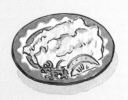

MAIN MEALS

To ensure that you receive all the nutrients essential to good health, it is important to eat a wide variety of meals. Following a diet plan should not mean restricting your food selection and need not limit your social life; these recipes adapt popular dishes from home and abroad to meet low-fat dietary guidelines and many are suitable for entertaining. Those who are not watching their weight can have larger portions and eat more accompaniments to the meal to satisfy their needs, while toddlers can enjoy the same food in smaller quantities or with slight adaptations.

Get used to using healthier cooking options. For example, meat can often be browned in a non-stick pan without the need for added fat. Mince can be browned in the same way and then drained, which removes about 40 per cent of the fat it started out with. If you are worried about meat drying out while you are grilling it, instead of brushing it with oil try marinading it first for added tenderness and flavour. When roasting meat or poultry, place it on a rack over the roasting tin so that the fat drains away from the meat. Leaving the skin on chicken helps to keep it moist while it cooks, but you can reduce the fat level significantly if you remove the skin before serving.

When cooking casseroles, you can make them healthier by using less meat and increasing the quantity of vegetables or adding pulses such as lentils. Onions can be softened in a little stock, wine or water rather than being fried. The overall fat level can be reduced by making the casserole in advance, then chilling it so that the fat will set on the surface and can then be removed.

RED PEPPER AND BASIL FRITTATA

182 cals, 7.5 g fat per serving
Serves 6

Frittata makes a delicious meal eaten hot or cold and this one is packed with vitamin C. The fat-free method used here of cooking onions down to a sweet, melting mass is useful for other recipes, particularly casseroles.

450 g/1 lb onions, thinly sliced
425 ml/15 fl oz vegetable stock
2 red peppers, quartered and deseeded
350 g/12 oz potatoes, peeled and cut into 1.25 cm/½ in cubes
6 large eggs
salt and freshly ground black pepper
15 g/½ oz fresh basil, shredded
1 tsp olive oil

- Heat a large non-stick frying pan over a moderate heat and add the onions. Allow them to colour and soften slightly, then pour in 300 ml/10 fl oz stock. Allow to bubble down, stirring occasionally.
- Meanwhile, grill the peppers until the skins are charred. Allow them to cool, then peel off and discard the skins and cut the peppers into thin strips. Cook the cubed potato in salted water for about 8 minutes or until tender. Drain and set aside.
- When the onion liquid has disappeared and the onions have browned a little, add half the remaining stock and allow it to bubble away and the onions to brown more. Repeat with the last of the stock. Allow the onions to cool and rinse the pan.
- Beat the eggs in a large bowl, season well with salt and pepper, then add the basil, peppers, potato and onions.
- Heat the oil in the frying pan and tip in the egg mixture. Cook over a low heat for 10 minutes until the underside is golden and the frittata is almost set. Place under a moderate grill until the top is set and golden. Leave to stand for 5 minutes. Turn out and serve with a mixed leaf salad.

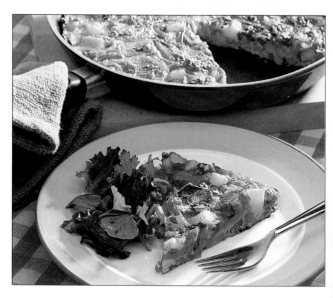

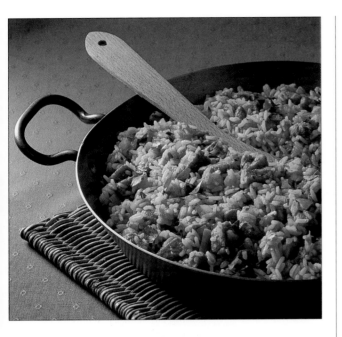

PORK PAELLA

434 cals, 12 g fat per serving
Serves 4

Traditionally, the Spanish dish paella is made with seafood or chicken but for a healthy change try using lean pork. It has only slightly more fat than skinless chicken and is a good source of protein, zinc and B vitamins, especially B$_{12}$.

1 tbsp corn oil
450 g/1 lb tenderloin of pork, cut into 1.25 cm/½ in cubes
1 large onion, chopped
2 cloves garlic, crushed
1 tsp paprika
½ tsp ground turmeric
400 g/14 oz can tomatoes, chopped
300 ml/10 fl oz chicken or vegetable stock
225 g/8 oz long grain rice
salt and freshly ground black pepper
1 tbsp chopped fresh parsley to garnish

■ Heat the oil in a non-stick wok or large, deep frying pan with a lid. Add the pork and fry until browned. Add the onion, garlic, paprika and turmeric and cook for a further few minutes. Add the tomatoes, stock and rice.
■ Cover and simmer for 20 minutes until the rice is cooked and all the liquid is absorbed. Stir frequently and check that the mixture is not sticking to the pan (if it is, add a little more liquid). Season to taste and garnish with the chopped parsley. Leave to stand for 5 minutes before serving.

MOROCCAN CHICKEN TAGINE WITH APRICOTS

335 cals, 9 g fat per serving
Serves 4

This fragrant stew features all the flavours of Middle Eastern cookery, where the combination of meat and fruit in one dish is quite common.

1 whole chicken (approximately 1.3 kg/3 lb), jointed into 8 pieces and skin removed, or a pack of 8 thighs and drumsticks
2 medium onions, finely chopped
2 cloves garlic, crushed
1 tbsp grated fresh ginger
pinch of saffron
¼ tsp ground turmeric
2 tsp ground cumin
2 tsp ground coriander
1 tsp ground cinnamon
salt and freshly ground black pepper
juice of 1 lemon
400 g/14 oz can chickpeas, rinsed and drained
115 g/4 oz no-soak dried apricots
2 tbsp chopped fresh coriander to garnish

■ Place the chicken joints in a tagine or flameproof casserole with the onion, garlic, fresh ginger, spices and plenty of seasoning. Mix together well, pour in the lemon juice then add enough cold water to just cover. Bring to a gentle simmer, cover with a lid and simmer very gently for 45 minutes.
■ Add the drained chickpeas and apricots to the casserole, stir into the liquid and simmer uncovered for a further 30 minutes.
■ When the cooking time is up, remove the chicken, chickpeas and apricots from the liquid and place in a warmed serving dish. Return the casserole to the heat and boil the liquid to reduce it by about a third. Pour the sauce over the chicken and scatter the coriander over before serving. Serve with plenty of couscous to soak up the delicious sauce.

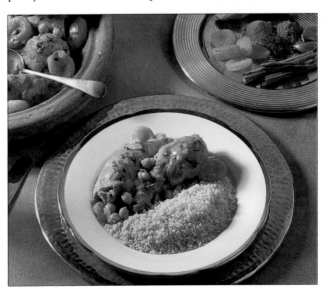

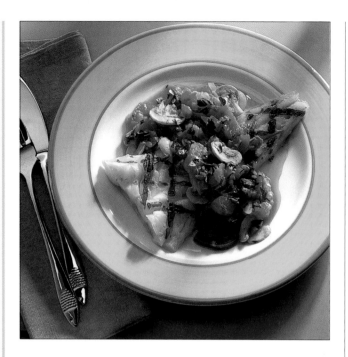

FISH CREOLE

198 cals, 4.5 g fat per serving
Serves 4

White fish, such as cod and haddock, is the perfect addition to a slimmer's diet. It has a low fat and calorie content but is high in protein.

1 onion, chopped
1 stick celery, chopped
115 g/4 oz mushrooms, sliced
1 small green pepper, deseeded and sliced
400 g/14 oz can chopped tomatoes in garlic
3 tbsp tomato purée
salt and freshly ground black pepper
pinch of chilli powder
dash of Tabasco sauce
1 tbsp olive oil
675 g/1½ lb cod or haddock fillets, skinned and cut
    into 4 pieces
1 tbsp chopped fresh parsley

■ In a large non-stick frying pan gently dry-fry the onion, celery, mushrooms and pepper for 10 minutes. Add the tomatoes, tomato purée, seasoning, chilli powder and Tabasco sauce. Simmer uncovered for 30 minutes until the vegetables are tender and the sauce has thickened.
■ Heat the oil in a ridged grill pan until it is slightly smoky. Place the fish in the pan and grill for 8–10 minutes, turning the fish once halfway through the cooking time (the fish should show the grill marks from the pan). Pour the sauce over the fish and serve garnished with chopped parsley.

WARM TERIYAKI CHICKEN WITH SESAME DRESSING

284 cals, 8 g fat per serving
Serves 4

The tangy marinade in this recipe keeps the meat moist and adds flavour. The vegetables are only cooked briefly so that they retain much of their vitamin content.

4 tbsp teriyaki sauce
1 tbsp clear honey
½ tsp Chinese five spice powder
4 boneless, skinless chicken breasts, about 150 g/5½ oz each
175 g/6 oz green beans, trimmed
175 g/6 oz sugar snap peas, trimmed
175 g/6 oz broccoli florets

For the dressing:
1 tbsp soy sauce
1 tbsp clear honey
½ tsp sesame oil
1 tbsp sesame seeds, toasted and crushed
1 red chilli, deseeded and finely chopped
6 spring onions, sliced

■ To make the marinade: mix together the teriyaki sauce, honey, and Chinese five spice powder. Put the chicken in a shallow dish and pour the marinade over. Cover and marinate for at least 30 minutes, turning occasionally.
■ Remove the chicken from the marinade and cook under a preheated grill for 15 minutes, or until cooked through, basting occasionally with the marinade to give a glossy finish.
■ Meanwhile, cook the green beans, sugar snap peas and broccoli florets in boiling salted water for 3 minutes.
■ For the dressing: whisk the soy sauce, honey and sesame oil together. Mix in the sesame seeds, chilli and spring onions.
■ Drain the vegetables, toss them in the dressing and arrange on plates. Slice the chicken and place on top of the vegetables. Serve with boiled rice or thread noodles.

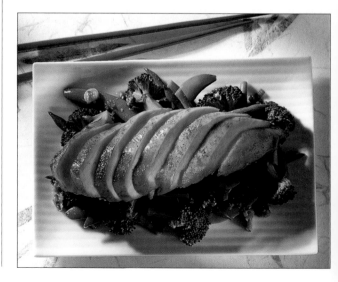

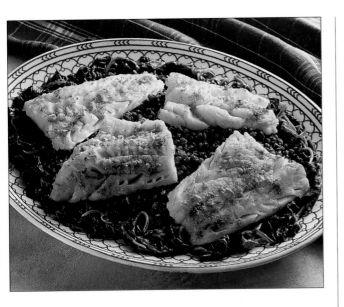

SPICED COD WITH PUY LENTILS

342 cals, 5.5 g fat per serving

Serves 4

Pulses are a good, economical source of protein and bulk out soups, burgers and stews. Puy lentils hold their texture when cooked and take up flavours well.

225 g/8 oz Puy lentils
2 tsp each ground cumin and coriander seeds
350–425 ml/12–15 fl oz vegetable stock
salt and freshly ground black pepper
½ tsp Chinese five spice powder
2.5 cm/1 in piece fresh ginger, grated
grated zest and juice of 1 lime
4 pieces cod fillet, each about 150 g/5½ oz, skinned
1 clove garlic, crushed
1 tsp olive oil, plus extra for greasing
450 g/1 lb young leaf spinach

■ Put the lentils into a saucepan, add half the cumin and coriander and 350 ml/12 fl oz of the stock. Season with pepper, but not salt as it stops the lentils cooking properly. Simmer, covered, over a gentle heat for 30–45 minutes until the liquid is absorbed and the lentils are tender. Check the lentils half way through the cooking time, adding more stock if needed.

■ Mix the remaining spices with the five spice powder, ginger, lime zest, half the lime juice and a little salt and pepper. Rub this paste into the cod fillets. Set aside.

■ When the lentils are almost cooked, place the cod fillets on a lightly oiled baking sheet and grill about 10 cm/4 in from moderate heat for 5–7 minutes (depending on thickness).

■ Meanwhile, sauté the garlic in the olive oil in a large pan. Gradually add the spinach, tossing it as it comes into contact with the heat, until it has just wilted. Season with salt and pepper. Stir the remaining lime juice into the lentils and check seasoning.

■ Serve the cod on a bed of the spinach and lentils.

COUNTRY CASSEROLE

233 cals, 8 g fat per serving

Serves 4

Light ale may seem an inappropriate ingredient for a calorie-controlled meal. Here, however, it gives good flavour and adds only 24 calories per portion.

1 tbsp olive oil
450 g/1 lb lean chuck steak or shin of beef, cut into large cubes
1 onion, sliced
2 carrots, sliced
1 clove garlic, crushed (optional)
115 g/4 oz mushrooms, wiped and sliced
300 ml/10 fl oz light ale
1 meat stock cube
1 tsp malt vinegar
1 tsp brown sugar
1 bay leaf
2 tsp cornflour
salt and freshly ground black pepper
1 tbsp chopped fresh parsley for garnish

■ Preheat the oven to 180°C/350°F/Gas mark 4. In a non-stick frying pan heat the oil and brown the meat on all sides. Transfer the meat to a 1.75 litre/3 pint casserole. Add the onion, carrots, garlic and mushrooms.

■ In a jug, blend together the light ale, stock cube, vinegar and brown sugar. Pour this mixture over the meat and vegetables and add the bay leaf. Cover and cook in the preheated oven for 1½–2 hours or until the meat is tender.

■ In a cup, blend the cornflour with 3 tbsp water then stir into the casserole. Return to the oven for a further 15 minutes for the gravy to thicken. Season to taste.

■ Serve piping hot garnished with the chopped parsley, and accompanied by fresh green vegetables and boiled potatoes.

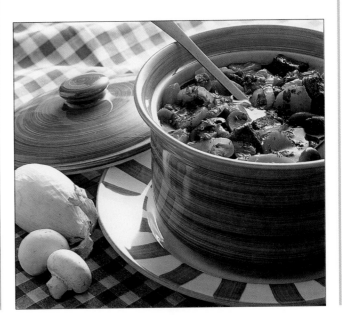

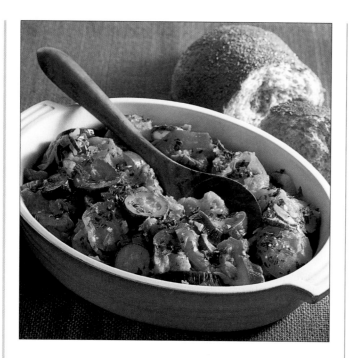

RATATOUILLE

110 cals, 4 g fat per serving
Serves 4

A dish that combines a variety of vegetables helps to ensure a balanced diet. This recipe offers a range of nutrients and is particularly rich in vitamin C.

1 large aubergine, about 350 g/12 oz cut into 2.5 cm/1 in slices
4 courgettes, about 225 g/8 oz, cut into 2.5 cm/1 in slices
1 tbsp oil
2 onions, chopped
2 cloves garlic, crushed
1 red pepper, deseeded and sliced into rings
1 green pepper, deseeded and sliced into rings
2 tbsp chopped fresh parsley
450 g/1 lb tomatoes, skinned and sliced
salt and freshly ground black pepper

■ Place the aubergine and courgettes in a colander, sprinkle with salt and press down with a plate; place heavy weights on top to hold. Leave for an hour and then rinse and pat dry with paper towels. While this stage is not essential, the flavour of the dish will be greatly enhanced by it.
■ Heat the oil in a pan, add the onion and garlic and cook gently for about 5 minutes. Add the peppers, aubergine and courgettes, and half the parsley. Cover the pan and simmer gently for 35 minutes until the vegetables are soft but retain their shape.
■ Stir in the tomato slices gently (try to keep the various foods intact), and simmer for about 10 minutes more with the lid off so that the tomato is heated through and the liquid reduced. Season with salt and pepper as necessary.
■ Place in a serving dish and sprinkle over the remaining parsley before serving.

FISH KEBABS WITH TARRAGON AND SESAME OIL SEASONING

140 cals, 4 g fat per serving
Serves 4

These kebabs made with pieces of cod provide a nutritious, low-calorie meal. For entertaining, in place of the cod you could use monkfish, shellfish, tiger prawns or scallops.

450 g/1 lb thick cod fillet, skinned and cut into
    2.5 cm/1 in cubes
1 medium green pepper, deseeded and cut into squares
    about 2.5 cm/1 in
4 firm tomatoes, cut into quarters
12 button mushrooms, wiped clean
8 bay leaves
16 seedless grapes
1 tbsp sesame oil for brushing
fresh lemon juice
2 tsp chopped fresh tarragon or 1 tsp dried tarragon

■ On a board, divide all the ingredients equally into four separate piles. To make the kebabs, thread the fish cubes and the different vegetable and fruit items in turn on to eight lightly greased skewers.
■ Brush the kebabs with the sesame oil. Sprinkle with plenty of lemon juice and tarragon.
■ Lay the kebabs on a baking tray. Cook under a moderately hot grill for about 15–20 minutes, turning frequently, until the fish and vegetables are cooked. Brush with the remaining oil and sprinkle with more lemon juice and tarragon each time they are turned.
■ Serve accompanied by fresh green vegetables in season or a salad, and boiled potatoes or rice.

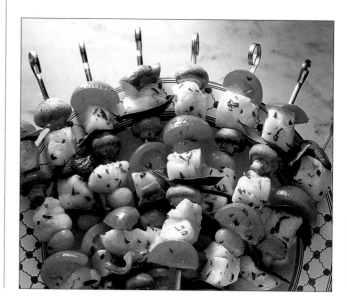

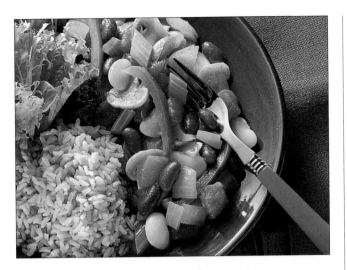

MIXED BEAN GOULASH

242 cals, 4.5 g fat per serving
Serves 4

This hearty goulash is an excellent low-fat source of protein and iron, especially important for people who don't eat meat.

115 g/4 oz butter beans
115 g/4 oz red kidney beans
1 tbsp corn oil
2 medium onions, chopped
2 sticks celery, chopped
115 g/4 oz mushrooms, wiped and sliced
1 medium green pepper, deseeded and sliced
1 tbsp paprika
400 g/14 oz can tomatoes, chopped

■ Soak both types of beans in a large bowl of water for 8–10 hours. Drain them, transfer to a large saucepan and cover with fresh cold water. Bring to the boil and boil rapidly for at least 10 minutes, skimming any scum from the surface. Lower the heat, cover and simmer for 40 minutes or until tender.
■ Meanwhile, heat the oil in a large flameproof casserole and fry the onion and celery for 3 minutes. Add the mushrooms and pepper and cook for 2 more minutes. Stir in the paprika and the tomatoes with their juice and 450 ml/16 fl oz water. Bring to the boil and stir well.
■ Drain the beans and add them to the casserole, cover, lower the heat and simmer for 30 minutes, stirring occasionally. Serve accompanied by brown rice and a green salad.

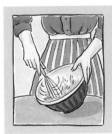

HEALTHY EATING TIP
Eaten with a grain food such as rice, kidney beans are a good source of fat-free protein. Red kidney beans are high in potassium and iron and also contain phosphorus, folate and zinc.

STUFFED AUBERGINES

289 cals, 9.5 g fat per serving
Serves 4

Native to India, the aubergine is becoming a popular vegetable and when baked is very low in calories. The addition of other vegetables and rice to this recipe increases protein and energy.

2 large aubergines, trimmed and cut in half lengthwise
2 tbsp corn oil
1 medium onion, finely chopped
1 stick celery, finely chopped
1 carrot, finely chopped
115 g/4 oz brown rice
2 cloves garlic, crushed (optional)
4 tbsp tomato purée
salt and freshly ground black pepper
55 g/2 oz fresh breadcrumbs
1 tbsp chopped fresh herbs
55 g/2 oz low-fat Cheddar cheese, grated

■ Preheat the oven to 180°C/350°F/Gas mark 4. Scoop out the flesh of the aubergines taking care not to break the shells, chop the flesh and put the shells aside. Heat the oil in a large pan and add the aubergine flesh, onion, celery, carrot and rice. Stir well together and fry for a few minutes. Add half the garlic and the tomato purée.
■ Cover with water and simmer for about 40 minutes until the rice and vegetables are cooked and the mixture has thickened. Season to taste with salt and pepper. Pile the mixture into the four aubergine shells.
■ Mix the breadcrumbs, herbs and remaining crushed garlic and sprinkle over the filled aubergine shells. Place the filled shells on a baking sheet and bake in the oven for 15 minutes.
■ Sprinkle the cheese over the breadcrumbed top and place the aubergines under a hot grill until the cheese melts and begins to turn golden. Serve hot accompanied by a green salad.

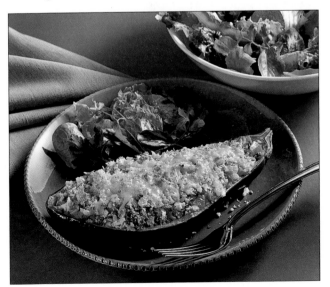

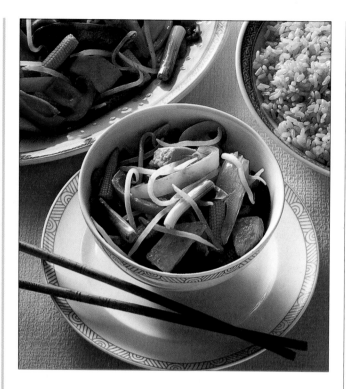

CHINESE CHICKEN

381 cals, 5.5 g per serving
Serves 4

The high protein and low fat value of the chicken in this recipe is complemented by the vegetable mixture which provides vitamins and other vital nutrients.

150 g/5 ½ oz uncooked brown rice
225 g/8 oz cooked chicken, skin removed
1 tsp corn oil
1 tsp grated root ginger
1 clove garlic, crushed
1 red and 1 yellow pepper, deseeded and sliced
115 g/4 oz mangetout
115 g/4 oz baby corn, cut into thirds
115 g/4 oz mushrooms, sliced
4 sticks celery, sliced
1 bunch spring onions, sliced in 4 cm/1½ inch lengths
115 g/4 oz beansprouts
2 tbsp soy sauce
4 tbsp dry sherry
salt and freshly ground black pepper

■ Put the rice on to cook. Cut the chicken into smallish pieces. Heat the oil in a wok, add the ginger and garlic and fry for 5 seconds. Add the peppers, mangetout, baby corn, mushrooms and celery to the wok and stir-fry for 2–3 minutes.
■ Add the chicken and cook for 2 minutes, then add the spring onions, beansprouts, soy sauce and sherry, and allow to bubble for about 1 minute. Season to taste.
■ Transfer to a warmed serving dish and serve accompanied by the boiled brown rice.

DEVILLED LAMB

382 cals, 24 g fat per serving
Serves 4

Lamb is high in protein, rich in B vitamins and is an excellent source of both zinc and iron. Ensure the cuts are lean to keep the fat and calorie content low. By frying the lamb with onions and celery you can seal it without having to add extra oil to the recipe.

8 neck of lamb cutlets or lean loin of lamb chops,
    about 1 kg/2¼ lb total
2 sticks celery, sliced
1 onion, chopped
2 medium tomatoes, sliced
2 tsp dry mustard
150 ml/5 fl oz stock
150 ml/5 fl oz dry red wine
1 tsp Worcestershire sauce
salt and freshly ground black pepper

■ Trim any visible fat from the lamb. Fry the cutlets in a non-stick pan with the celery and onion until they are brown and the surface of the meat is sealed. Place the tomatoes over the meat in the pan.
■ In a measuring jug, mix the mustard to a paste with a little of the stock, then add the rest of the stock, the red wine and the Worcestershire sauce. Stir together well then pour over the meat and bring to the boil.
■ Preheat the oven to 180°C/350°F/Gas mark 4. Transfer the lamb and other ingredients to a large casserole, cover and cook for approximately 1½ hours or until the meat is cooked and beginning to come away from the bone. Season to taste.
■ Allow the casserole to cool, skim any fat that has risen to the surface and then reheat.
■ Serve with mashed potatoes and fresh vegetables in season.

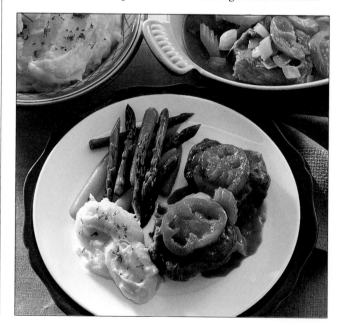

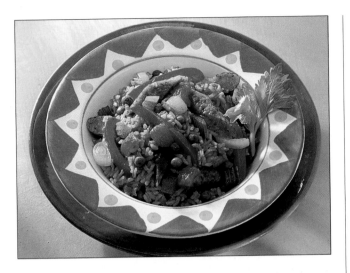

JAMBALAYA

448 cals, 14 g fat per serving
Serves 4

This spicy Spanish-Creole dish is rich in nutrients and fibre. Sausages are used for taste but to lower the fat content you could use skinless chicken instead.

1 tsp corn oil
1 medium onion, chopped
1 stick celery, chopped
½ red pepper, deseeded and cut into strips
1 clove garlic, chopped
1 tsp chilli powder
225 g/8 oz long grain brown rice
450 ml/16 fl oz chicken stock
400 g/14 oz can chopped tomatoes
450 g/1 lb low-fat sausages, grilled and cut into chunks
75 g/2¾ oz frozen peas
3 drops Tabasco sauce
salt and freshly ground black pepper

■ Heat the oil in a large pan and fry the onion, celery and pepper without letting them brown. Stir in the garlic, chilli powder and rice. Cook until the rice is opaque. Add the stock and tomatoes. Bring to the boil, reduce the heat and simmer.
■ When the rice is nearly cooked, add the sausage chunks to the pan along with the frozen peas and Tabasco sauce.
■ Continue to cook for a further 10 minutes or until the peas and sausage are heated through thoroughly and the liquid is fully absorbed. Add salt and pepper to taste.

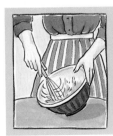

HEALTHY EATING TIP
As rice is gluten-free it is safe for people with wheat intolerance. Because brown rice goes through only minimal milling, it contains a greater amount of vitamins, minerals and fibre than white rice.

SMOKED HADDOCK *EN PAPILLOTE* WITH TOMATO SALSA

156 cals, 1.5 g fat per serving
Serves 4

Baking en papillote *(in a paper parcel) keeps the food moist, as all the juices are sealed in. Here, the salsa is a tasty fat-free alternative to traditional butter sauces.*

450 g/1 lb ripe tomatoes
½ red onion, very finely chopped
½ red pepper, deseeded and very finely chopped
½ red chilli, deseeded and very finely chopped
grated zest and juice of 1 lime
salt and freshly ground black pepper
4 pieces of smoked haddock fillet, each about 150 g/5½ oz
115 g/4 oz asparagus tips (or sugar snaps or green beans)

■ For the salsa: place the tomatoes in a bowl, pour boiling water over them and leave them for a few moments. Remove from the boiling water with a slotted spoon and cool in a bowl of cold water for a few minutes. Peel off the skins and discard. On a chopping board, quarter the tomatoes; remove and discard the seeds, then chop finely. Mix with the onion, pepper, chilli, lime zest and juice. Season and leave to stand.
■ Meanwhile preheat the oven to 220°C /425°F/Gas mark 7.
■ Cut out four 38 cm/15 in diameter circles of greaseproof paper, fold in half to crease and then open out. Brush lightly with a little oil. Place a piece of fish to one side of the crease of each paper circle. Spoon some salsa on top of the fish, and divide the asparagus tips between the parcels. Seal the parcels by pleating (folding) around the edges. Chill the remaining salsa.
■ Place the parcels on baking sheets and bake for 12 minutes.
■ Serve the parcels unopened, for your guests to fully savour the aroma as they tear open the paper. Serve the reserved salsa separately for a hot/cold contrast.

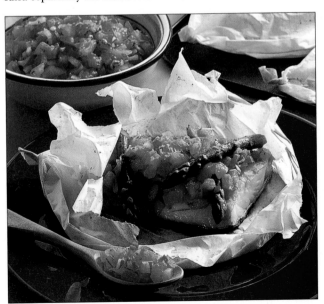

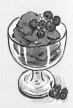

DESSERTS

Hidden fat and sugar in recipes and ready-made desserts can often be the downfall of a weight control plan. But being on a diet doesn't mean you have to forgo desserts altogether – by making your own desserts you can control your calorie and fat content.

Because it is completely fat-free, one of the most suitable foods to eat for dessert is fresh fruit. Although some taste very sweet, such as ripe summer fruits like peaches and strawberries, the sugar content is from natural (intrinsic) sugars. Choose fruits which you can happily eat without added sugar. For example, pink grapefruit has a natural sweetness whereas ordinary grapefruit is very tart. Be careful with tinned fruits as they are often preserved in calorie-laden syrup; look instead for those that are packed in their own juice. Topping your fruit with low-fat yoghurt instead of cream or ice-cream is an easy way to cut back on calories.

Yoghurt is a quick and nutritious dessert in its own right. The range available varies hugely in calorie and fat content so check the label and try to go for low-fat, low-sugar varieties.

This section gives you the opportunity to try a variety of delicious desserts and still stick to a healthy and calorie-controlled diet. As you will see most recipes will work with less sugar than most recipe books suggest (except for meringue). Adding dried fruit will often sweeten cakes and puddings so that they need no sugar, or at least less than they would normally, as well as increasing the fibre content. Flavourings such as cinnamon, cloves, vanilla, grated fresh ginger and orange zest have a sweetening effect. Ready-made apple purée can be used to add moisture (and sweetness) without fat in cake recipes, or you can soak dried fruit overnight in tea, then add as much of the soaking liquid as you need to make a fruit cake without adding any fat at all.

EXOTIC FRUITS

Delicious exotic or unusual fruits are becoming more widely available and can add nutritious variety to your diet. These fruits can be served on their own as a dessert or may be added to a fruit salad.

PAPAYA

Cut in half from top to bottom and scoop out the seeds. Cut into slices like a melon and sprinkle lemon juice over, or cut into chunks and serve in fruit salads.
Per 100 g: 36 calories, trace fat

PASSION FRUIT

Cut in half around the middle, scoop out the aromatic yellow, juicy pulp and eat it with a teaspoon. The seeds are eaten, not discarded. It is delicious added to fruit punch and can also be used to add flavour to fruit pies.
Per 100 g: 36 calories, 0.5 g fat

LYCHEE

Serve as a dessert fruit on its own or add to fruit salad. Pinch the outer skin to crack it, then peel it off. Discard the stone. The flesh is white and juicy with a delicate flavour.
Per 100 g: 58 calories, trace fat

MANGO

Do not prepare until just before serving. Cut the fruit lengthways, peel the skin back with a knife and scoop out the pulp with a spoon. The orange/yellow flesh is very juicy with a delicate fragrance and taste.
Per 100 g: 57 calories, trace fat

KIWI FRUIT

Cut in half around the middle and scoop out the pulp with a teaspoon in the same way you would eat a boiled egg. Alternatively, peel carefully and cut into slices. Add to fruit salads or use to decorate various puddings.
Per 100 g: 49 calories, 0.5 g fat

FIGS

Remove the stalk and slice in half lengthways. The skin and flesh can be eaten as can the seeds and the sweet pulp.
Per 100 g: 43 calories, trace fat

GUAVA

Cut in half and scoop out the flesh with a teaspoon. The seeds should be eaten. Can be enjoyed raw or baked.
Per 100 g: 26 calories, 0.5 g fat

POMEGRANATE

Cut in half across the middle like a grapefruit and use a teaspoon to prise out the sections. Eat the seeds.
Per 100 g: 51 calories, trace fat

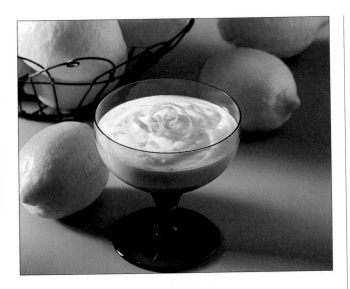

SYLLABUB

69 cals, 0.5 g fat per serving
Serves 4

This light and tangy dish is traditionally made with cream but yoghurt makes a very healthy low-fat alternative and adds protein and calcium to the diet.

1 unwaxed lemon
300 g/10½ oz low-fat natural yoghurt
2 tbsp white wine
2 tbsp fresh lemon juice
honey to taste

- Pare off a few fine strips of lemon rind and reserve to garnish the finished dish, then grate the rest. In a bowl, blend together the yoghurt, wine, lemon juice and grated rind and stir to form a smooth mixture.
- Add honey to taste.
- Spoon into four sundae dishes or standard size wine glasses and chill for at least an hour. Garnish each with a little lemon rind just before serving.

DAILY MEAL PLAN

BREAKFAST: Oat, Fruit and Nut Muesli (page 133); 330 ml/11 fl oz fresh orange juice
MID-MORNING SNACK: Nectarine
LUNCH: Tiger Prawn Fajitas with Salsa (page 134); glass of mineral water
DINNER: Red Pepper and Basil Frittata (page 142) served with Crunchy Salad with Vinaigrette (page 139); glass of mineral water
DESSERT: Syllabub; herbal tea

TOTAL FOR THE DAY: 1519 calories, 38 g fat

SUMMER FRUIT ROULADE

189 cals, 5.5 g fat per serving
Serves 6

Summer berries are not only delicious but also rich in vitamin C. The Greek yoghurt adds a rich, creamy taste. For a lower-calorie dessert, use low-fat yoghurt.

3 large eggs
85 g/3 oz castor sugar
grated zest of 1 orange
85 g/3 oz plain flour, sifted
pinch of salt
115 g/4 oz Greek yoghurt
350 g/12 oz mixed summer berries
a little castor sugar or icing sugar to dust

- Line a 20 x 30 cm/8 x 12 in Swiss roll tin with non-stick baking parchment before you start to make the cake. Preheat the oven to 190°C/375°F/Gas mark 5.
- Put the eggs, castor sugar and orange zest in a large bowl and whisk with an electric whisk until the mixture is pale and mousse-like, and the beaters leave a thick trail.
- Sift the flour and salt over the mixture and quickly and carefully fold in, using a large metal spoon. Be careful not to knock too much air out of the mixture. Pour into the Swiss roll tin, and shake gently to distribute the mixture evenly.
- Bake on the centre shelf of the oven for 12–15 minutes or until the sponge is golden and springy to the touch.
- Remove from the oven and turn out on to a sheet of baking parchment. Carefully peel away the base paper then start to roll up the roulade and parchment from the short side. Leave to cool wrapped in the parchment.
- When you are ready to serve the roulade, gently unroll the sponge, spread with the Greek yoghurt and scatter the berries over evenly.
- Roll up the roulade, lifting away the paper as you roll. Dust the roulade with a little castor sugar or icing sugar.

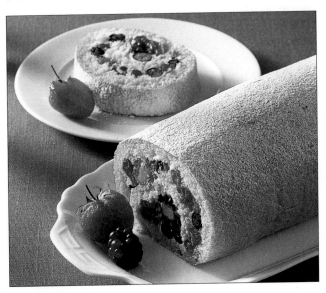

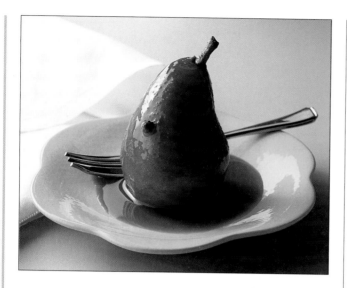

PEARS IN RED WINE

188 cals, trace fat per serving

Serves 4

Pears provide a useful source of fibre, vitamin C and potassium. The addition of red wine or cider makes this a flavoursome dessert.

4 large firm ripe pears (such as Comice)
55 g/2 oz castor sugar
300 ml/10 fl oz red wine
1 tsp fresh lemon juice
2 cinnamon sticks
½ tsp arrowroot
4 cloves

■ Peel the pears, keeping them whole with stalks attached. Place the sugar, wine, lemon juice and cinnamon sticks in a saucepan and boil until it reduces a little. Blend the arrowroot with 1 tbsp cold water and add to the mixture to thicken.
■ Lay the pears in a saucepan and stick a clove into each one. Pour the wine mixture over the pears, cover and simmer gently for 25–30 minutes or until the pears are just tender when tested with the point of a sharp knife. Turn the pears once during cooking to ensure even colouring. Remove the pears carefully with a slotted spoon and transfer to a large serving dish or four individual dishes.
■ Remove the cloves and cinnamon sticks. Boil the remaining liquid until it is reduced and thickened and pour over the pears. Serve warm or chilled.

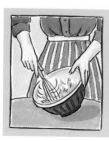

HEALTHY EATING TIP

If you would prefer to serve an alcohol-free dessert, use grape juice instead of red wine for the pears. This reduces the energy content as grape juice has less than half the calories of red wine.

FRUIT SALAD FOOL

176 cals, 1 g fat per serving

Serves 4

Dried fruit is high in fibre and is a concentrated source of nutrients, especially iron and potassium. Use any mix that suits your taste, but avoid using prunes in this dessert as they will discolour it.

225 g/8 oz mixed dried fruit such as peaches, apricots, pears and apples
tea made with 1 fruit or Earl Grey teabag
1 banana, peeled
juice of half a lemon
225 g/8 oz low-fat natural yoghurt
a few drops of almond essence to taste (optional)

■ From the mixed fruit, put aside three dried apricots. Place the remaining dried fruit in a bowl, cover with cold Earl Grey tea or fruit tea and soak for at least 12 hours for maximum flavour.
■ Transfer the soaked fruit and liquid to a saucepan and stew gently until tender, about 15 minutes. Drain the fruit well and place with the banana and the lemon juice in a liquidiser. Purée till smooth then pass through a sieve to remove any fibres. Place the puréed fruit in a large bowl and fold in the yoghurt. Taste for sweetness and add a few drops of almond essence if desired.
■ Divide equally between four dessert dishes or tall glasses. Chop the reserved apricots and use to garnish. Keep refrigerated until just before serving.

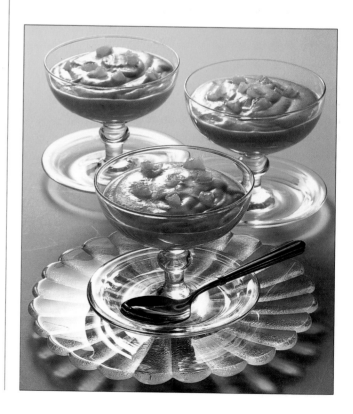

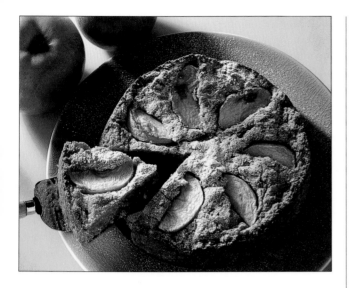

APPLE CAKE

267 cals, 12.5 g fat per serving

Serves 8

Cake is one food that dieters feel they should forgo, but here is a healthy alternative to high-calorie shop-bought products.

225 g/8 oz wholemeal flour, sifted
2 tsp baking powder
1 tsp ground cinnamon
1 tsp ground cloves
115 g/4 oz polyunsaturated margarine
115 g/4 oz brown sugar
400 g/14 oz cooking apples, peeled and cored

■ Preheat the oven to 190°C/375°F/Gas mark 5. In a bowl, stir together the flour, baking powder and spices then rub in the fat until it resembles breadcrumbs. Stir in the sugar. Put aside half an apple and grate the remainder; stir it into the mixture.

■ Place the mixture in a lightly greased 19 cm /7½ in round tin. Cut the reserved apple into wedges and arrange these on the top. Bake for 35 minutes or until a knife put into the cake comes out clean and the top is brown and crispy.

DAILY MEAL PLAN

BREAKFAST: Menu 4 (page 132)
MID-MORNING SNACK: Orange
LUNCH: Scrambled Eggs with Smoked Salmon and Cottage Cheese (page 140); mineral water
DINNER: Warm Teriyaki Chicken with Sesame Dressing (page 144); green salad; glass of fresh fruit juice
DESSERT: Apple Cake; cup of herbal tea

TOTAL FOR THE DAY: 1760 calories, 61 g fat

MELON SURPRISE

109 cals, 0.5 g fat per serving

Serves 4

This versatile fruit dish is low in calories and contains beta-carotene and vitamin C. The mixture of fruits ensures a variety of textures and colours that will delight both the palate and the eye.

4 small canteloupe melons
1 pink grapefruit
1 large orange
1 kiwi fruit
115 g/4 oz white seedless grapes
a few strawberries and mint leaves to garnish

■ Carefully cut off the tops of the melons and keep them to one side. Scoop out the seeds with a teaspoon. Use a ball cutter to remove the melon flesh, taking care not to pierce the sides. Reserve the melon balls and juice in a bowl.

■ Cut the grapefruit and orange into segments taking care to remove all skin and pith. Cut the segments in half and add to the melon balls.

■ Peel the kiwi fruit, cut into slices, cut the slices in half and add with the grapes to the melon and citrus fruit.

■ Mix all the fruit together taking care not to break up the pieces. Leave the bowl of fruit in the refrigerator to chill for at least an hour before serving.

■ Divide the fruit mixture equally between the four melon shells, which make attractive serving dishes, then pour the juices over, and decorate with one or two strawberries and mint leaves. Replace the reserved top of each melon just before serving.

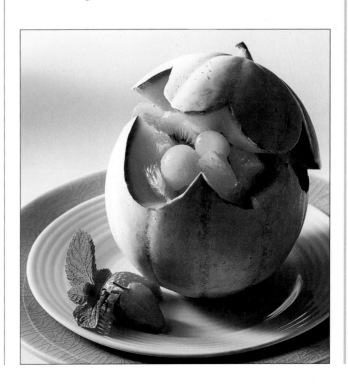

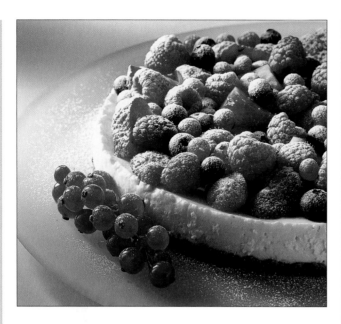

LEMON BERRY CHEESECAKE

224 cals, 7.5 g fat per serving
Serves 8

*Many dieters find cheesecake a terrible temptation.
This reduced fat version, however, will not pile on the
kilos and is packed with healthy summer fruits.*

115 g/4 oz ginger snap biscuits, crushed
25 g/1 oz low-fat margarine, melted
grated zest and juice of 2 lemons
11 g/¼ oz sachet powdered gelatine
2 x 250 g/9 oz tubs Quark
200 g/7 oz Greek yoghurt
2 large egg yolks
70 g/2½ oz castor sugar
450 g/1 lb mixed berries, such as strawberries, blueberries,
   raspberries and redcurrants
icing sugar to dust

■ Preheat the oven to 160°C/325°F/Gas mark 3. Mix together
the crushed ginger snaps and melted margarine, and press
into the base of a 20 cm/8 in loose-based cake or flan tin.
Bake in the oven for 10 minutes or until hard to the touch.
■ Place 3 tbsp of the lemon juice in a small heatproof bowl
and sprinkle the gelatine over.
■ Leave to stand for 5 minutes, then place the bowl in a
saucepan of barely simmering water and leave until the
gelatine has completely dissolved.
■ Place the Quark, Greek yoghurt, egg yolks, castor sugar and
remaining lemon juice and zest in a food processor and blend
until smooth. Gradually pour in the clear gelatine through a
strainer and quickly process to blend in.
■ Pour the mixture over the base, cover and chill for at least
3 hours until set.
■ To serve, pile on the berries and dust with icing sugar.

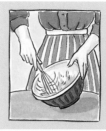

HEALTHY EATING TIP

Egg whites contain very little of the
cholesterol and saturated fat of whole
eggs. This makes desserts such as
sorbets, which don't use the yolk, a
good option for slimmers.

RASPBERRY WATER ICE

45 cals, trace fat per serving
Serves 4

*Raspberries are both delicious and nutritious, being
rich in vitamin C. This dessert provides an excellent
low-fat and low-calorie alternative to ice cream.*

225 g/8 oz raspberries
25 g/1 oz icing sugar
425 ml/15 fl oz diet lemonade
2 egg whites
mint leaves for garnish

■ Reserve a few raspberries for garnish, then place the rest
together with the icing sugar in a liquidiser and blend to a
purée. Add lemonade to make up to 425 ml/15 fl oz. Transfer
the mixture to a plastic container, cover with a lid or foil
and place in the freezing compartment of a refrigerator.
■ When the mixture begins to set around the side of the
container, scrape this away with a fork and gently stir it into
the centre of the container. This should break up the ice
crystals. Whip the egg whites until stiff and fold them into the
raspberry mixture. Cover the container, return it to the freezer
compartment and leave until set.
■ To serve, divide equally between four glass dishes or dessert
bowls – use an ice cream scoop if desired. Garnish with the
reserved raspberries and mint leaves.

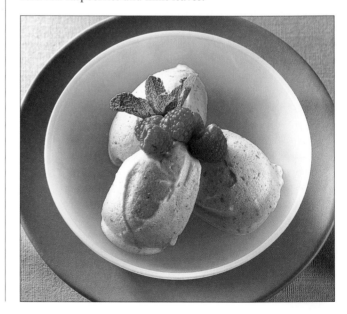

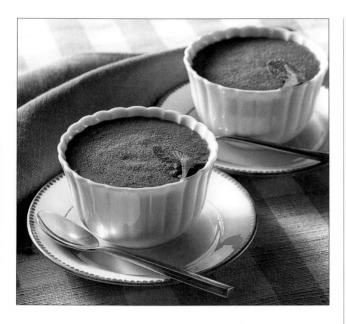

CHOCOLATE CREAM

84 cals, 0.5 g fat per serving
Serves 4

Using low-fat fromage frais in place of cream in this dessert makes it surprisingly low in calories. Use good quality drinking chocolate to add useful minerals.

250 g/9 oz low-fat fromage frais
40 g/1½ oz drinking chocolate powder (not cocoa)
2 tsp castor sugar
6 drops vanilla essence
4 sprigs of fresh mint to garnish

■ Beat all the ingredients together in a bowl until all the chocolate powder is evenly blended and the mixture is creamy and smooth.
■ Divide the mixture equally between four dessert dishes with a capacity of 100 ml/3½ fl oz each.
■ To decorate, sprinkle the surface of each cream very lightly with a little more drinking chocolate powder and add a sprig of mint. Refrigerate until ready to serve.

DAILY MEAL PLAN

BREAKFAST: Menu 3 (page 132)
MID-MORNING SNACK: 20 g/¾ oz blueberries with 100 g/3½ oz low-fat yoghurt
LUNCH: Chicken Tikka Pittas (page 141) with fresh salad and 2 slices of wholemeal bread; mineral water
DINNER: Country Casserole (page 145) with boiled carrots and 2 wholemeal rolls; glass of fresh fruit juice
DESSERT: Chocolate Cream; herbal tea

TOTAL FOR THE DAY: 1468 calories, 26 g fat

BAKED STUFFED APPLES WITH CUSTARD

270 cals, 0.5 g fat per serving
Serves 4

The high fructose content of apples helps to control blood sugar level and the vitamin C content boosts the immune system. Custard is an ideal accompaniment adding protein and calcium.

4 Bramley cooking apples (or other), about 225 g/8 oz each
115 g/4 oz sultanas
4 tbsp water
4 cloves

For the custard:
600 ml/1 pint skimmed milk
2 tbsp custard powder
castor sugar to taste

■ Preheat the oven to 190°C/375°F/Gas mark 5. Wipe the apples well and remove the cores with an apple corer. Make a shallow cut through the skin around the middle of each apple. Stand them in an ovenproof dish, so that they fit tight enough to stay upright during cooking.
■ Stuff the centre of each apple with the sultanas and put 4 tbsp water in the bottom of the dish. Push two cloves into the skin of each apple. Bake for about 30 minutes or until the apples are cooked right through.
■ To make the custard, place 4 tbsp of the milk into a cup or small bowl. Heat the remaining milk in a saucepan. Meanwhile blend the custard powder with the reserved milk until it forms a smooth paste. Gradually add this to the milk in the pan and bring to the boil, stirring until the custard thickens. Add castor sugar to taste as required.

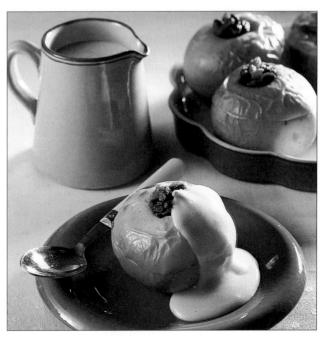

155

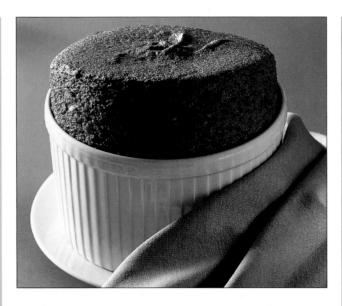

BLACKCURRANT SOUFFLÉ

92 cals, trace fat per serving
Serves 4

This handsome dessert is strong on flavour and rich in vitamin C – weight for weight, blackcurrants contain four times as much of this vitamin as an orange.

450 g/1 lb blackcurrants (or other flavoursome fruit)
55 g/2 oz sugar
4 egg whites, whipped until stiff

■ Preheat the oven to 190°C/375°F/Gas mark 5. Wash the blackcurrants, remove any stems and transfer to a pan. Add the sugar and stew in a very small amount of water until cooked, about 15–20 minutes.
■ Sieve the fruit or blend in a food processor until it is thick and smooth (it should make about 300 ml/10 fl oz purée).
■ Carefully fold the purée into the egg whites so that it is well mixed yet all the air is retained.
■ Transfer the mixture to a lightly greased 18 cm/7 in soufflé dish and bake for 25 minutes until it is well risen and brown on top. Serve immediately.

DAILY MEAL PLAN

BREAKFAST: Menu 4 (page 132)
MID-MORNING SNACK: Peach
LUNCH: Mediterranean Tomato Soup (page 135) with 2 wholemeal bread rolls; glass of mineral water
DINNER: Fish Kebabs and Ratatouille (page 146) and 150 g/5½ oz boiled potatoes; glass of fruit juice
DESSERT: Blackcurrant Soufflé; cup of herbal tea or glass of mineral water

TOTAL FOR THE DAY: 1208 calories, 25.5 g fat

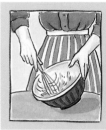

HEALTHY EATING TIP

If you prefer not to cook with gelatine you can substitute either agar agar, a type of seaweed, or arrowroot. Read the labels to determine how much you need to replace the gelatine.

COEUR À LA CRÈME

155 cals, 4 g fat per serving
Serves 4

The fat-reduced dairy products on supermarket shelves today allow the full nutritional benefits of dairy food to be enjoyed without adding too many calories. Dairy foods are rich in protein, calcium and vitamin B$_{12}$.

350 g/12 oz cottage cheese, sieved or liquidised till smooth
150 g/5½ oz low-fat natural yoghurt
juice of half a lemon
2 tsp gelatine
6 apricots
12 strawberries to garnish

■ In a bowl combine the cottage cheese, yoghurt and lemon juice. Soak the gelatine in 2 tbsp of cold water in a cup for 5 minutes. Place the cup in a pan of simmering water until the gelatine is dissolved; gradually stir into the cheese mixture.
■ Divide between four heart-shaped moulds with a capacity of 100 ml/3½ fl oz and leave in the refrigerator for 24 hours.
■ Before serving, chop the apricots (removing and discarding the stones) and liquidise with 1 tbsp water to the consistency of a smooth purée. Carefully turn out the creams from the moulds onto individual plates; pour a little of the puréed fruit over each and garnish with the fresh strawberries.

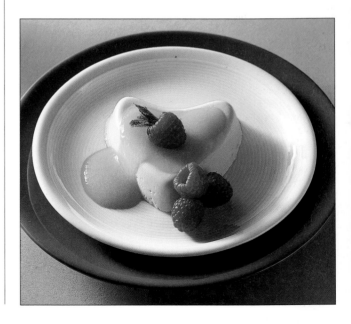

INDEX

ACKNOWLEDGMENTS

Carroll & Brown Limited
would like to thank
British Dietetics Association
British Food and Drink Federation
Penny Hunking, Energise, Surrey
Tessa Prior, Infant & Dietetics Food
    Association, London
The Pritikin Longevity Centre
Slimming World
Tesco Stores
Weight Watchers UK and Weight
    Watchers International, Inc,
    New York, USA
Wendy Doyle, Nutritionist

Editorial assistance
Richard Emerson
Sharon Freed
Simon Warmer

Design assistance
Simon Daley
Mari Hughes
Matt Sanderman

Photograph sources
8 Rex Features/Tim Rooke
9 Courtesy of The Pritikin
    Longevity Centre
10 Image Bank/David De Lossy
11 Popperfoto
12 Science Photo Library/Prof. P.
    Motta/Dept. of anatomy/
    university 'La Sapienza', Rome
16 National Gallery, London/
    Bridgeman Art Library, London
17 (Top) Helsinki City Museum's
    Photographic Archive, (Bottom)
    Pictorial Press
19 The National Trust Photo Library
20 Zefa-Stockmarket
22 Tony Stone Worldwide/David
    Madison

29 Images Colour Library
35 (Bottom) Tony Stone
    Images/Dennis O'Clair
36 Science Photo Library/Oscar
    Burriel
41 Courtesy of Professor Fairburn
43 Corbis-Bettmann
46 Hutchison Library/Lesley Melson
47 Tony Stone Images/Philip &
    Karen Smith
54 Images Colour Library
58 Angela Hampton/Family Life
    Pictures
61 Tony Stone Images/Jon Gray
62 Tony Stone Images/Nick Dolding
78 Tony Stone Images/David
    Madison
85 John Walmsley
88 Private Collection/Bridgeman Art
    Library, London
92 Courtesy of the National College
    of Naturopathic Medicine,
    Portland, Oregon, US
94 World View/Igno
    Cuypers/Science Photo Library
95 Tony Stone Images/Christopher
    Bissell
97 (Top) Explorer/JL Charmet,
    (Bottom) Wellcome Institute,
    London
98 Novosti/Bridgeman Art Library,
    London
100 (Top) Pictorial Press Limited,
    (Bottom) The Hutchison
    Library/Errington
101 Tony Stone Images/Leland Bobbe
112 Tony Stone Images/Christopher
    Bissell
113 Russ Capps, photographer
114 Courtesy of Weight Watchers
    International, Inc
116 Tony Stone Images/Lori A. Peek
119 Tony Stone Images/Doug Armand

Medical illustrators
Sandie Hill
Paul Williams

Illustrators
Victor Ambrus
Janie Coath
Lorraine Harrison
Bill Piggins
Christine Pilsworth
Sarah Venus

Photographic assistants
M-A Hugo
Mark Langridge

Hair and make-up
Rachel Atwood
Bettina Graham
Kym Menzies

Picture researcher
Sandra Schneider

Food preparation
Maddalena Bastianelli
Eric Treuillé

Research
Steven Chong

Index
Steven Chong
Laura Price

Note
Metric and imperial measures are given throughout except when calculating
measures of nutrients, which are given in metric only. Calorie and fat contents
for foods and recipes are a guide only as it is not possible to give precise figures.

75·006·01

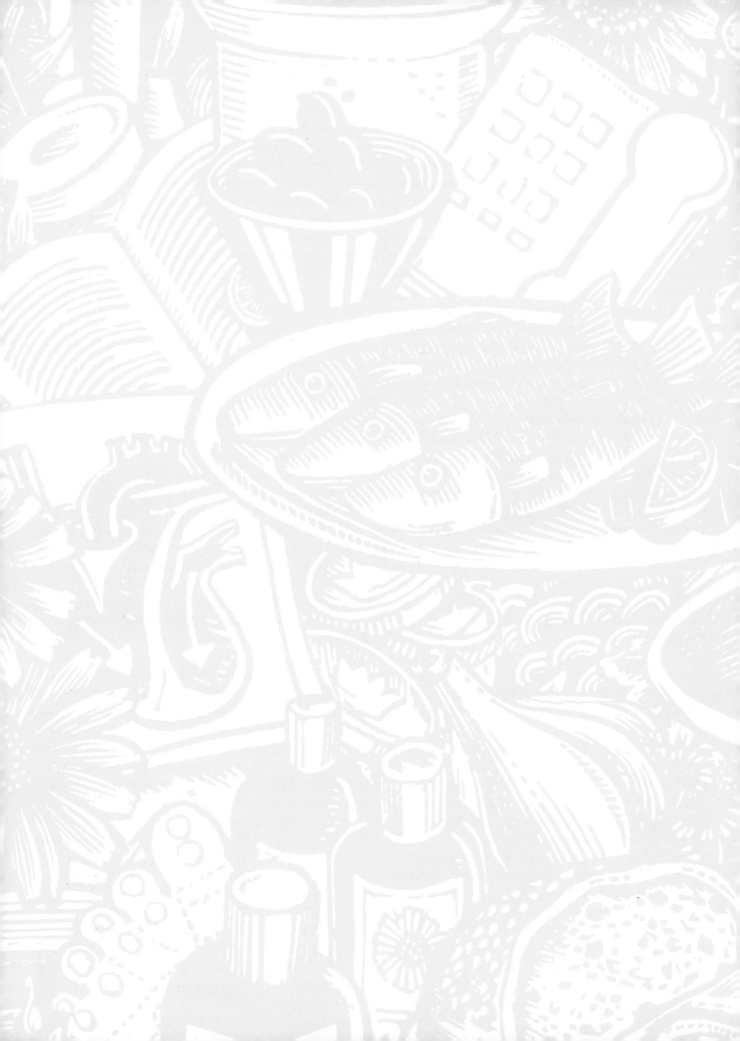